# I AM FEA███████SS

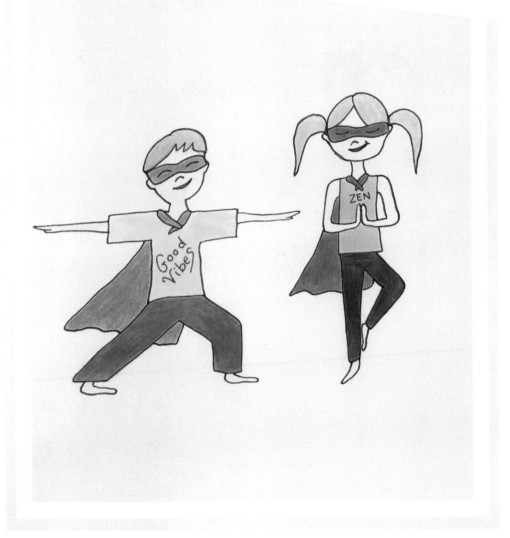

## A Yoga Story for Kids
## and Superheroes

Library of Congress Cataloging-in-Publication Data Available

ISBN: 978-1-7751434-2-0

Published by Art Mindfulness and Creativity
www.artmindfulnessandcreativity.com

Dedicated to our two
little Yogi's

KAI AND ELLA

# Mountain Pose

Standing with my feet planted and pressing to the ground, eyes closed, gazing in, palms open forward, feel the strength of a mountain flowing through your body.

You are Fearless.

When I feel afraid, I take a deep breath and stand tall against what scares me.

# I AM FEARLESS

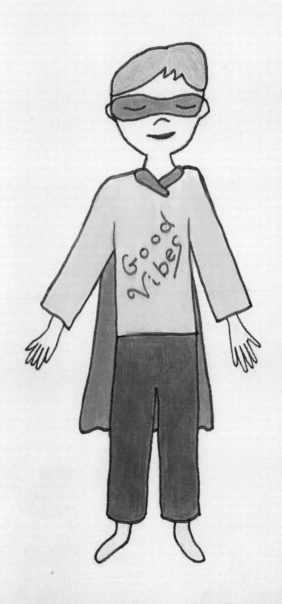

## Chair Pose

Inhale your arms shoulder height, growing tall and proud through your upper body, take a sinking bend into your knees as you grow powerful towards the earth and the sky.

You are Strength.

When I feel powerless in a situation, I remind myself how strong my body and mind really are.

# I AM STRENGTH

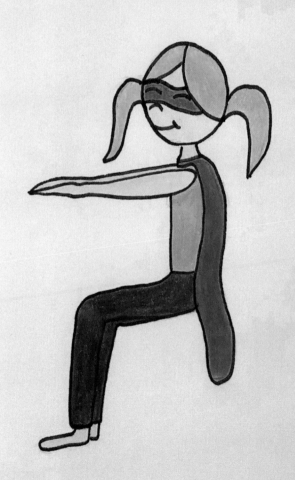

# DRINKING BIRD

Trust your body as you lean forward and become a free bird. Lifting high onto your toes, remember how strong you can become, as you squeeze your legs together and feel power through the torso. You are Free.

When I feel trapped, I fly into each moment with confidence like a bird.

I AM FREE

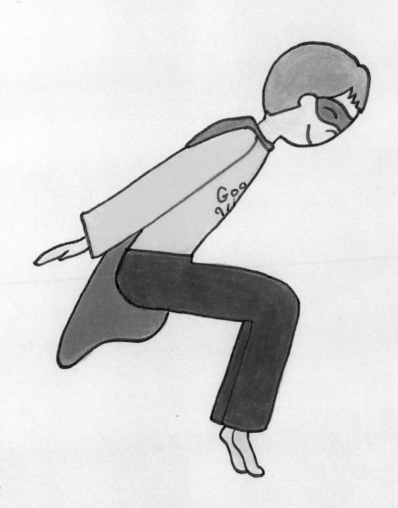

# WARRIOR

I take the stance of the warrior, feeling both feet growing roots, raising arms high above, take the stance of battle as you breathe in.

You are a Warrior.

When I am faced with hard times I ground my feet with determination and conquer the situation.

# I AM A WARRIOR

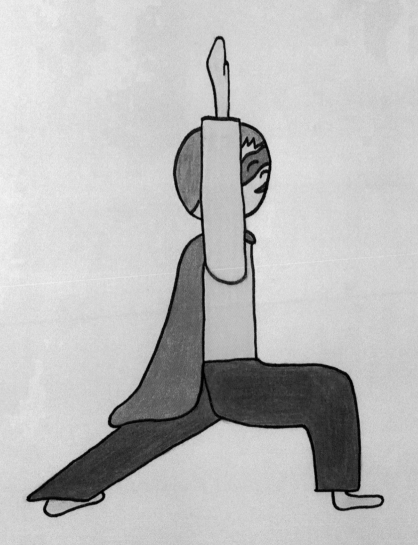

# AIRPLANE

Trust in your grounded leg to lift and fly, reaching
arms out with purpose and grace, rising up,
you float into the air.
You are Balanced.

When I am unsure, I lift up my spirit and soar, finding harmony, even in the most shaky situations.

# I AM BALANCED

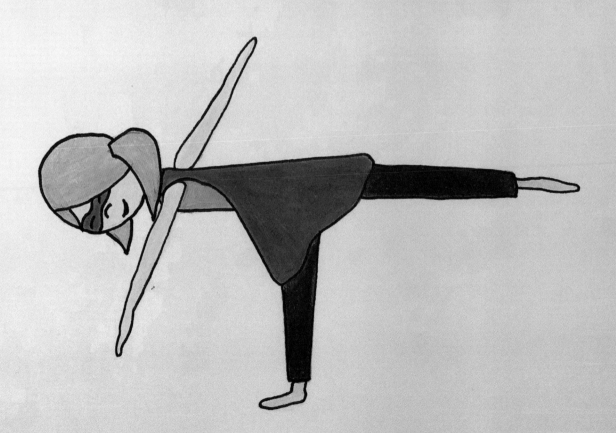

# Half Moon

Maintain trust in the balance and strength you have already gained as you stack your body so you can fit between two panes of glass. One hand to ground you down, one to lift yourself high.

You are Abundant.

I remind myself daily how loved and cared for I am. My heart and spirit are full.

# I AM ABUNDANT

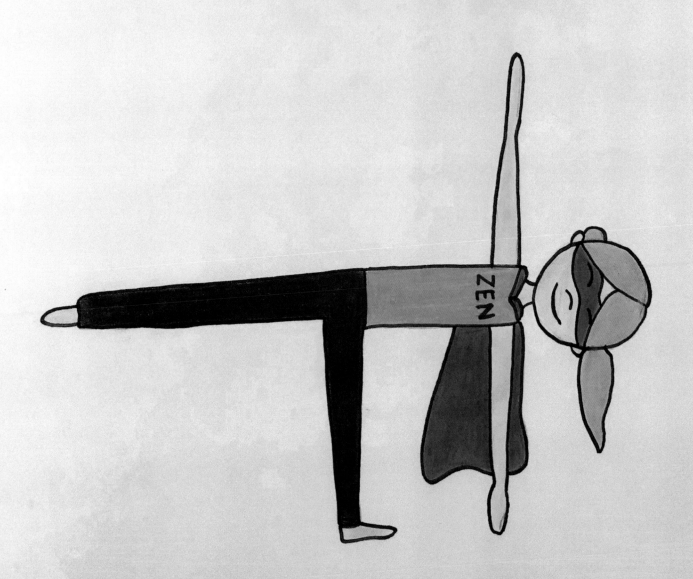

## ARROW

Push into the earth and fill yourself with strong breath as you lift into your arrow, feeling the energy fill your core, you rise up.
You are Powerful.

When I am feeling like a failure, I can take a deep breath and point myself in the direction I want to go.

# I AM POWERFUL

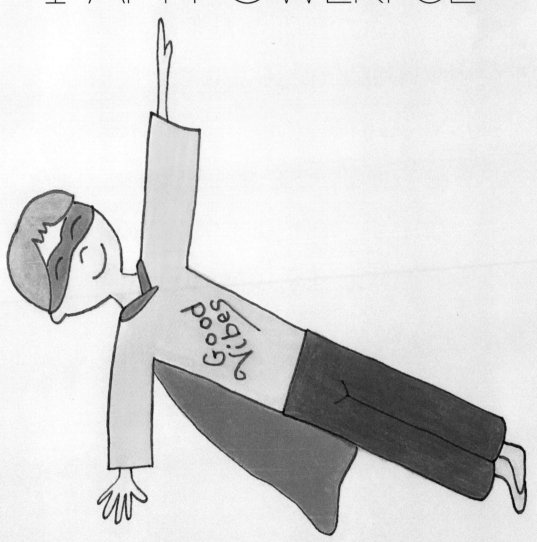

# Yogi Squat

Exhale and descend to the earth into a yogi squat, feeling connected to the energy here, close your eyes and place your palms together and in front of your heart.

You are Grounded.

When life feels overwhelming, I can calm myself
down, focusing on calm deep breathes, settling
back to the earth.
I AM GROUNDED

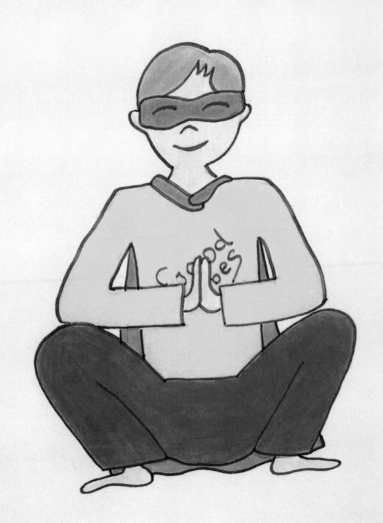

# DANCER'S

Grabbing onto your ankle and tipping forward,
reaching to the stars feeling adventurous,
trust in your body.
You are Graceful.

When life feels messy and clumsy, I feel the ground beneath me and grasp firmly with my toes, so I can grow tall and secure, reminding myself of the playful and fun side of life.

I AM GRACEFUL

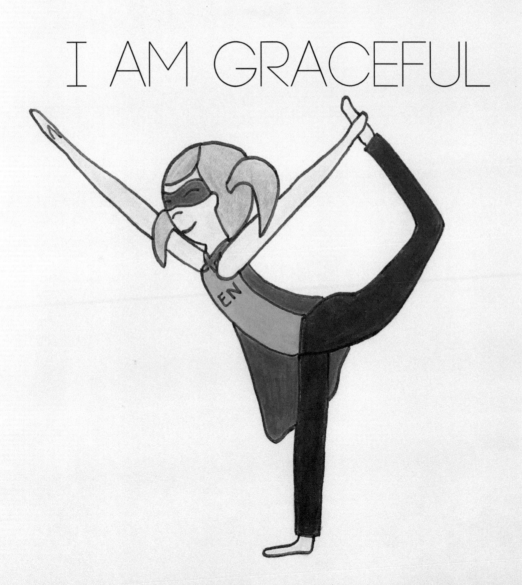

# GODDESS

Legs and arms wide, squatting down, bend into
your lower body, knees wide, and stretching
high to the planets above.
You are Centered.

When my universe starts to feel shaky, I tune into my inner power and my heart to find the balance I need.

# I AM CENTERED

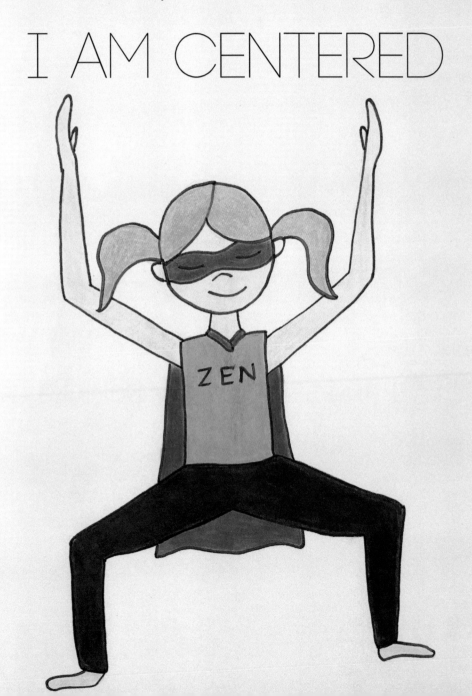

# MONKEY POSE

Trusting in your body, breath and mind to make you strong, you secure your hands, and the center of your head into a triangle shape and slowly take your knees onto the back of your arms, breathe and find steady slow balance here.
You are Brave.

I remind myself that when I feel fearful, I am full of superhero, and connect to the thought that I am capable of anything and everything.

I AM BRAVE

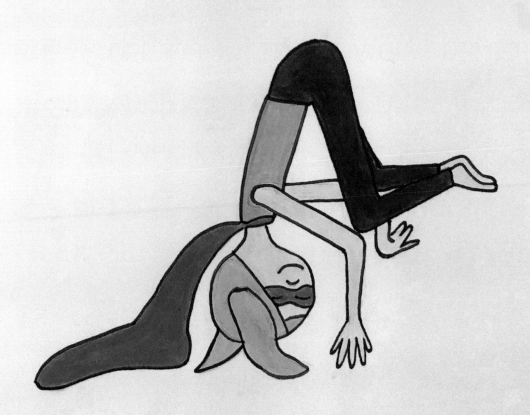

PARTNER DOWN DOG

When your friend takes this simple triangle shape called " Downward facing dog" , Slowly walk your feet up their back as you walk your hands back towards them. Eventually resting your feet gently on their low backs. Trust in each other.

You are Courage.

When meeting new people makes me nervous, or unsure, I remember to put faith in new connections and friends.

# I AM COURAGE

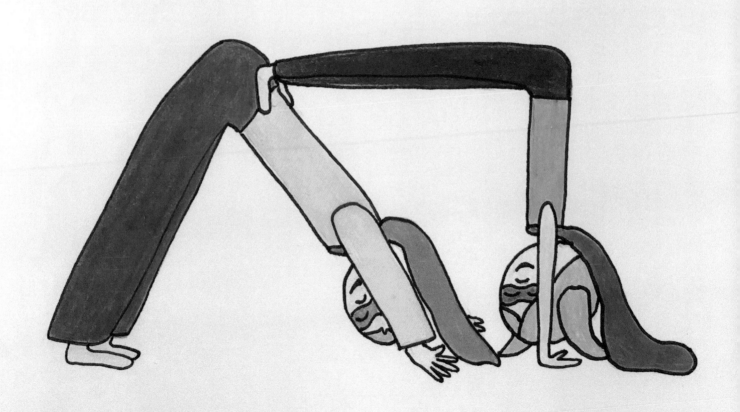

# PARTNER HEART OPENER

Back to back, hold hands with your partner. As you both breathe out, start to lean forward, open your heart centre to the sky.

You are Caring.

My heart is open and I have enough love to share with everyone around me, especially those who are in need of a helping heart.

I AM CARING

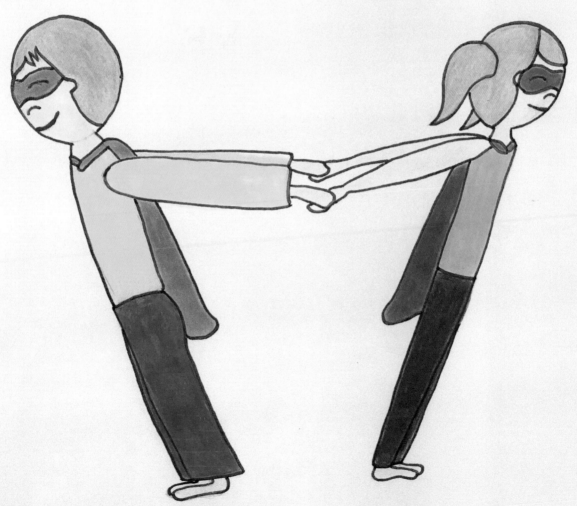

PARTNER BOAT

Using the strength and balance from your partner,
connect your feet together, lift your heart towards the
infinite sky, straighten your legs and smile from the
human connection. float there in strength.

You are Connected.

I am never alone, I always have someone to turn to, someone to listen to me, someone who cares about me.

# I AM CONNECTED

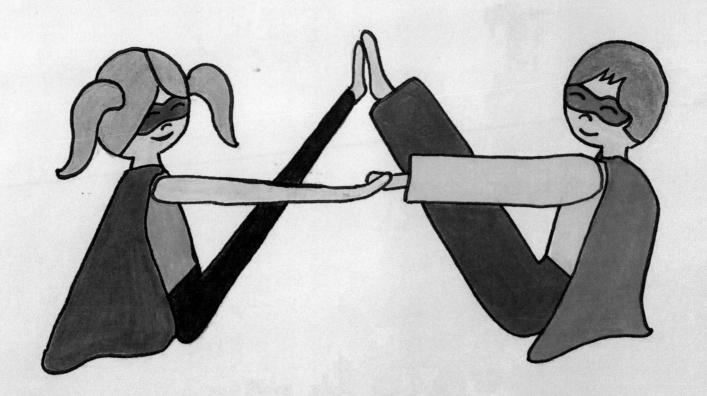

# LIZARD ON A ROCK

As your partner curls up into " Childs Pose" with knees tucked underneath them and forehead on the floor, gently start to lay your spine along their spine, connecting to each other.

Opening your arms and heart.

You are Enough.

I can be open to being a rock for someone when they need the extra support, I trust in my strength, and that when I need someone they will have my back too.

# I AM ENOUGH

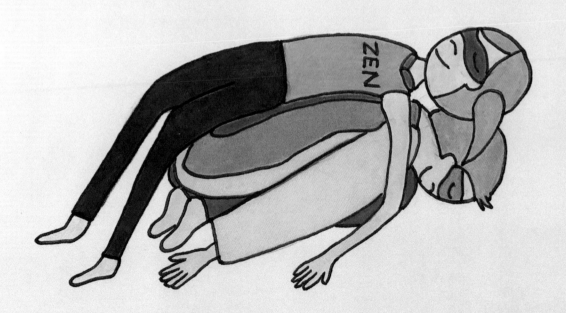

STACKED CHILD'S POSE

With yourself in child's pose, have your partner
softly lay in a hugging embraced child's pose
on top of yours.

Close your eyes and breathe together.

You are Supportive.

I can be the foundation for my friends and family. I am there for them when they need me to be. Open arms, open ears, open heart.

# I AM SUPPORTIVE

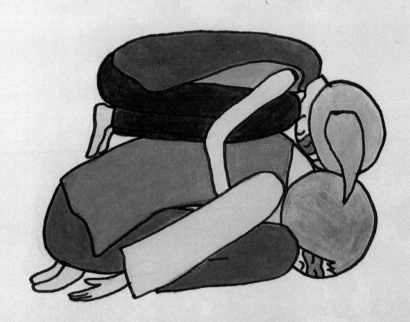

# BABY BRIDGE

Firmly press into your hands and feet as you lift your hips high. Pressing your heart through your open shoulders, opening yourself to all the good. You are Grateful.

When I feel down, I feel the beauty of life, and how it's filled with so many amazing people, so much health, and so much love. I rise up to happiness.

I AM GRATEFUL

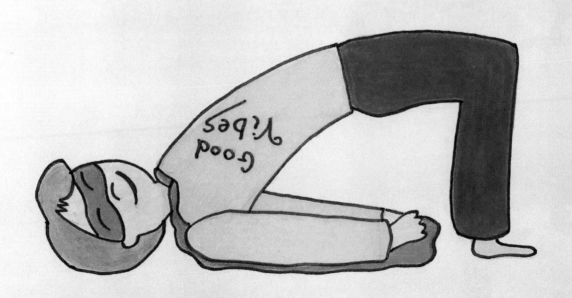

## CAMEL

From your knees, take your hands on your low back and lift your chest to the sky as you start to lean back into your camel pose. Let your head fall gently back as you open the light beam from your heart.

You are Radiant.

When I feel gloomy or dark, I remember the light from my heart, and how it shines on my entire body when I let the love flow. My heart beams and glows as I enter a room.

I AM RADIANT

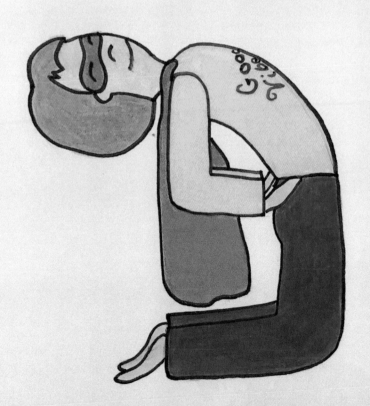

## FORWARD FOLD

Let your breath go as you melt towards your
legs, feeling length through your upper body,
connecting your belly to your legs.
This forward fold feels like a hug.
You are Whole.

When I feel empty, or sad, I remember I am filled
to the brim with love from everyone around me.

I AM WHOLE

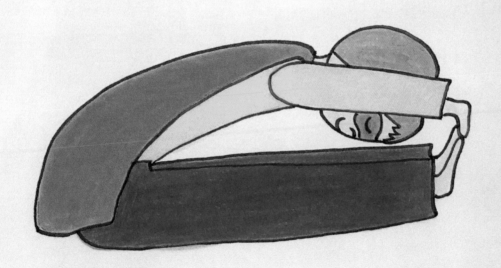

# BUMBLE BEE BREATH

Sit with your eyes closed, take a deep breath in, all the way to the bottom of your belly. When you exhale the breath through your nose, start to hum along with the exhale.

The exhale of your inner voice calms you.

You are Breath.

When I start to feel anxious and nervous, I can connect myself to my breath, and slow down with the guidance of inhales and exhales.

I AM BREATH

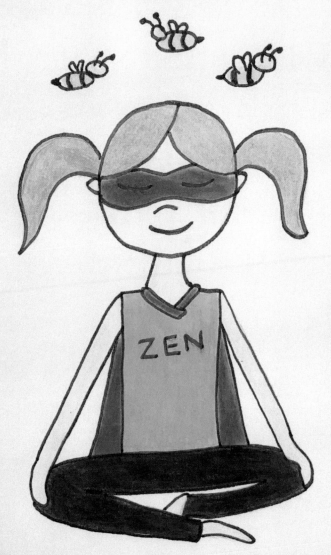

MEDITATIVE SEAT

Feel your body full of breath, strength and mental
calm as you open yourself to everything, and
allow the breath to
calm the stormy waters inside.
You are Peace.

When I feel angry or worked up, I can remind myself of my inner calm and soothe myself with the inner guide of my mind.

I AM PEACE

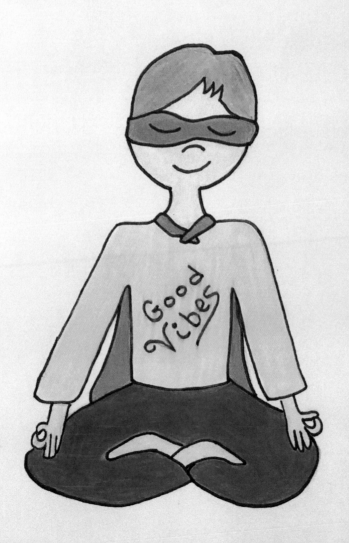

# SAVASANA

Laying yourself down, arms wide, legs wide, palms open, heart lifted, and eyes closed. The breath is calm, and the body and mind follow. These moments are for drifting and reconnection to yourself.

You are Divine Light.

And when the world seems chaotic, I can rest easy knowing I am light to myself, and to everyone around me. I am fearless, whole, strength, free, a warrior, balanced, abundant, powerful, grounded, graceful, centered, brave, courage, enough, caring, connected, supportive, grateful, radiant, breath, and peace.

I AM DIVINE LIGHT

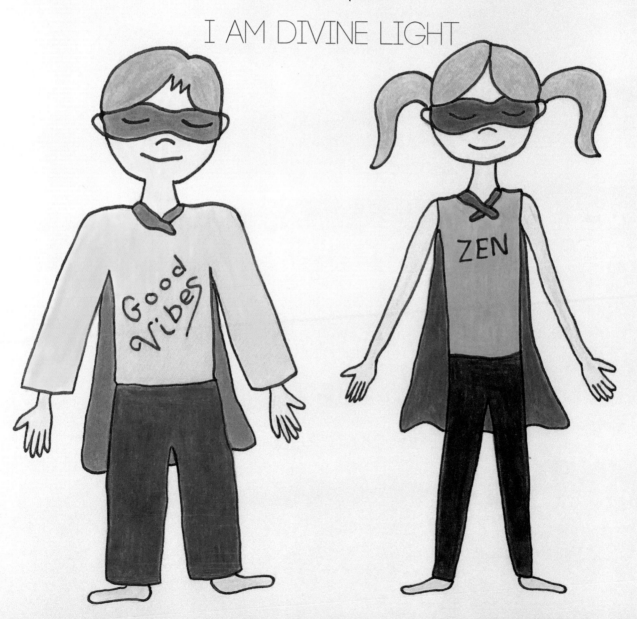

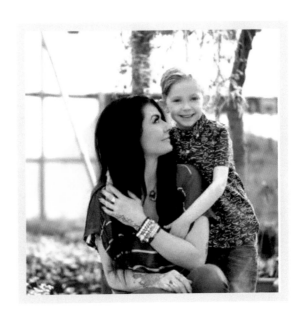

Apryl is a yoga teacher, writer and designer in Calgary, Alberta. She aspires to share her passions through creative expression, as she runs her own jewelry design business Apryl Dawn Designs, and has co-authored an Amazon #1 best selling book on thriving as an entrepreneurial mom boss.

www.apryldawn.com

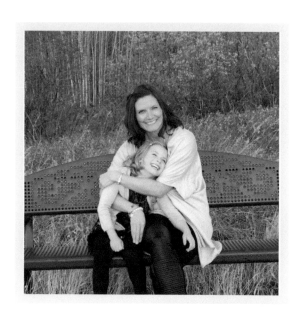

Believe, Create, Inspire

Mission is to help people develop and explore their creative gifts through art, yoga and mindfulness.

Amanda is an author, illustrator, and teacher (B.A, B.Ed, M.Ed). She lives in Calgary, Alberta with her daughter Ella

www.artmindfulnessandcreativity.com

# I PRACTICE YOGA

## What is your Super Power?

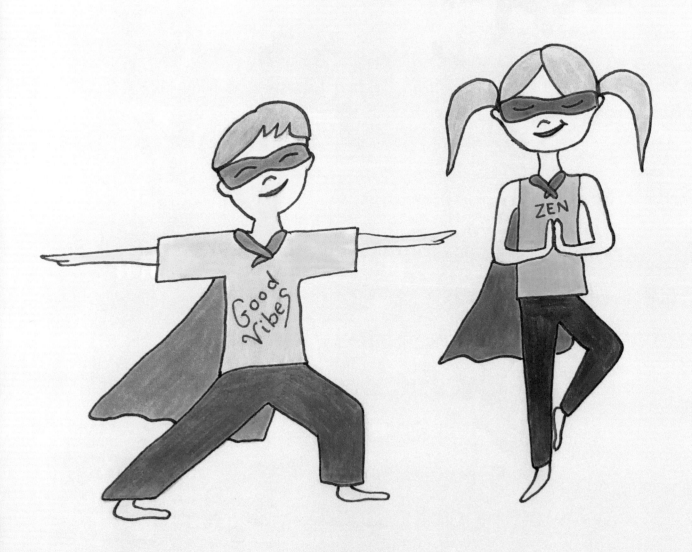

Printed in Great Britain
by Amazon

# Longman Practice Exam Papers

# A-level Pure Mathematics and Statistics

**Cyril Moss**
**Michael Kenwood**

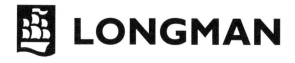 LONGMAN

Series editors:

## Geoff Black and Stuart Wall

## Titles available for A-Level
Biology

Business Studies

Chemistry

Physics

Psychology

Pure Mathematics and Mechanics

Pure Mathematics and Statistics

Addison Wesley Longman Limited
Edinburgh Gate, Harlow
Essex CM20 2JE, England
*and Associated Companies throughout the World*

First published 1999

ISBN 0-582-36925-8

British Library Cataloguing in Publication Data
A catalogue record for this book is available from the British Library

Set in Times 11/13 and Gill Sans by 38

Printed in Singapore by Addison Wesley Longman China Ltd, Hong Kong

# Contents

# How to use this book

In this collection of eight practice exam papers we have covered the work required for the Advanced Level and Advanced Supplementary Level in Mathematics. There are four practice papers containing questions on Pure Mathematics and four containing questions on Statistics. The syllabuses for different examination boards vary slightly in content and emphasis, so in these practice exam papers you may find the occasional question on a topic you have not met. You should check with your teachers and colleagues whether such a topic is part of your syllabus or not. Any question on a topic which is not included in your syllabus should be omitted when you work the practice paper, but this should not happen very often.

We have not tried to copy the pattern of the examination papers set by any one examination board. The practice papers here are all of two hours' duration, with no choice of questions. These practice papers are equally suitable for you whether you are taking a modular course or a linear course. Do not worry if you find that you need further time to complete a paper – as you practice each day, you will find that your rate will improve quite dramatically, as will your confidence. The solutions to the questions are given at the end of the practice papers. We have provided you with full solutions and an indication of how marks are earned as you build up the solution. Use the solutions positively, but always try to complete the whole paper first. These solutions are intended to help you to reach your full potential by the time you sit the examination. The mark schemes are included so that you can appreciate how marks are awarded. The three main types of marks used by examiners are as follows.

- **Method marks (M)** are awarded when you know a relevant method and use it.

- **Accuracy marks (A)** are dependent on the relevant method mark(s) being scored before accuracy marks are awarded. Accuracy marks are awarded for correct answers and also for correct answers being given despite an earlier error.

- **Independent marks (B)** are awarded for isolated correct answers or correct statements, and are not dependent on any method marks.

Many students tend to underachieve in the first A-level Maths examination paper they sit. To avoid this problem, sit a practice paper a few days before the 'real thing' and get rid of the nerves and inhibitions before the time when it really matters.

Here are a few more tips on good examination practice that we recommend.

- Make sure you have all the equipment you will need: paper on which to write your answers, pencil, pen, rubber, ruler, protractor, calculator (with either new or spare battery).

- Each board gives details in each question of the worth in terms of marks of the whole question and its parts. This gives you a clear message about how much time you should need to solve each question or part-question.

- Most papers start with the shorter questions and build up to the longer, structured ones. Papers are set so that questions are printed in increasing mark order. Experience over many years suggests that the best strategy for tackling papers in which there is no choice of questions is to solve the questions in the order set. However, do NOT spend too much time on any particular question; if you get stuck, leave the question and return to it later if you have time. Never cross anything out until you are sure that you have replaced the work with something better – let the examiner decide if your work deserves credit or not.

■ Wherever possible, use freehand sketch diagrams to supplement your written solutions. Draw accurate graphs only when the question specifically requires you to do so.

■ When you have completed a solution always read through the question again to ensure that you have given the final answers as the examiner demands. Many marks are lost by failing to notice this simple requirement.

■ Use ALL of the time allotted in the examination, even though you may think you have answered everything well before the end. Use any time left over to check your answers carefully.

■ NEVER spend time writing out the actual questions set by the examiner – the examiner knows what they are!

■ In longer questions with several parts, you are often asked to show that a result is true in the first part. If you cannot do this do not despair – assume the result is true and write a solution to the rest of the question based on this assumption. This is a common technique used by examiners to give all candidates the same starting point for the later stages of a structured question, when some of them may be unable to complete the first part. Everyone then has the same opportunity to gain all the available marks for the remainder of the question.

## Grades

The following guidelines should give you an indication as to how your efforts will affect the grade you receive in your A-level Mathematics exam. Each board has its own methods of grading, but, based on these practice exam papers, you can grade yourself as below and this will give a good indication of the grade you can expect to achieve in the real examination.

| | | | |
|---|---|---|---|
| **Grade A** | 80 marks and over | **Grade D** | 50–59 marks |
| **Grade B** | 70–79 marks | **Grade E** | 40–49 marks |
| **Grade C** | 60–69 marks | **Grade N** | 30–39 marks |

# Editors' preface

**Longman Practice Exam Papers** are written by experienced A-level examiners and teachers. They will provide you with an ideal opportunity to practice under exam-type conditions before your actual school or college mocks or before the A-level examination itself. As well as becoming familiar with the vital skill of pacing yourself through a whole exam paper, you can check your answers against examiner solutions and mark schemes to assess the level you have reached.

**Longman Practice Exam Papers** can be used alongside *Longman A-level Study Guides* and *Longman Exam Practice Kits* to provide a comprehensive range of home study support as you prepare to take your A-level in each subject covered.

# Acknowledgements

We record our appreciation and thanks to Tim Hills, Godalming Sixth Form College, and the Mathematics Department at Queen Elizabeth School for Boys, Barnet, who checked all the Statistics solutions.

Cyril Moss
Michael Kenwood

# Longman
## Examination Board

**General Certificate of Education**

**Pure Mathematics and Statistics**

**Paper 1 (Pure Mathematics)**

**Time: 2 hours**

**Instructions**

- Answer all questions.

- Make sure your method is clear, with sufficient working to show how the answer has been obtained.

| Number | Mark |
|--------|------|
| 1. | |
| 2. | |
| 3. | |
| 4. | |
| 5. | |
| 6. | |
| 7. | |
| 8. | |
| 9. | |
| 10. | |
| 11. | |
| 12. | |
| 13. | |
| 14. | |
| Total: | |

**Information for candidates**

- The number of marks is given in brackets at the end of each question or part-question.

- This paper has 14 questions. The maximum mark for this paper is 100.

---

1.  Solve the equation $27(3^x) = 9^{3x}$. **(3 marks)**

2.  The function f is defined for real values of $x$ by

    $$\text{f}: x \mapsto \frac{x-3}{2x-4}, \qquad x \neq 2.$$

    Find, in a similar form, the inverse function $\text{f}^{-1}$ of f. **(4 marks)**

3.  The three lines with equations $x + 2y = 3$, $2x + y = 1$ and $\lambda x + 3y = 4$ meet in the point $A$.

    Find the coordinates of $A$ and the value of the constant $\lambda$. **(5 marks)**

4.  $$\text{f}(x) \equiv 5x^3 + Ax^2 - 8x + 4,$$

    where $A$ is a constant.

    Given that $(x - 2)$ is a factor of $\text{f}(x)$,

    (a)  find the value of $A$, **(2 marks)**

    (b)  factorise $\text{f}(x)$ completely. **(3 marks)**

5.  Given that $0 < x < \pi$ and $y > 0$, find in its simplest form the solution of the differential equation $\dfrac{\mathrm{d}y}{\mathrm{d}x} = y \cot x$ for which $y = 2$ at $x = \dfrac{\pi}{6}$. **(5 marks)**

**Turn over**

1

**6.** The first and thirteenth terms of a geometric series are 16 and 2 respectively.

Find the sum to infinity of the series, giving your answer to 4 significant figures.

**(5 marks)**

**7.** The points $R$ and $S$ have position vectors $24\mathbf{i} + 7\mathbf{j}$ and $15\mathbf{i} + 20\mathbf{j}$ respectively, referred to an origin $O$.

(a) Show that $|\overrightarrow{OR}| = |\overrightarrow{OS}|$. **(2 marks)**

(b) By first finding the size of $\angle ROS$, find the size of $\angle ORS$, giving your answer to $0.1°$. **(4 marks)**

**8.**

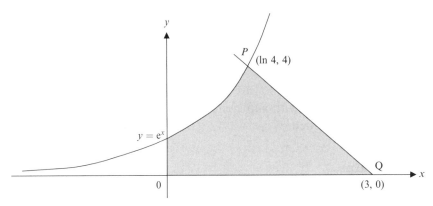

The point $P$ $(\ln 4, 4)$ lies on the curve $y = e^x$ and the line $PQ$ is such that $Q$ has coordinates $(3, 0)$, as shown. Find, giving answers to 3 significant figures,

(a) the gradient of the line $PQ$, **(2 marks)**

(b) the area of the shaded region. **(5 marks)**

**9.** A curve $C$ has equation $y^3 + 2xy^2 = 16$.

(a) Find $\dfrac{dy}{dx}$ in terms of $x$ and $y$. **(4 marks)**

(b) At the point $P$ on $C$, $y = -2$. Find the equation of the tangent to $C$ at $P$. **(3 marks)**

**10.** The curve $y = A\sin x + B\cos x$ passes through the points $\left(\dfrac{\pi}{4}, \sqrt{2}\right)$ and $(0, -3)$.

(a) Find the values of $A$ and $B$. **(4 marks)**

(b) Using your values of $A$ and $B$, find to 2 decimal places the two smallest positive values of $x$ for which $y = 0$. **(4 marks)**

**11.** A particle $P$ moves along a straight line so that its velocity $V\,\text{ms}^{-1}$ at time $t$ seconds after leaving a fixed point $O$ on the line is given by

$$V = 2t^2 - 3t + 4.$$

Find

(a) the acceleration of $P$ when $t = 4$, **(2 marks)**

(b) the distance which $P$ moves through between the instants when $t = 1\tfrac{1}{2}$ and $t = 3$, **(4 marks)**

(c) the minimum speed of $P$. **(3 marks)**

**12.** A curve is given parametrically by the equations

$$x = (1 + t)^2, \qquad y = (1 - t)^2, \qquad t \in \mathbb{R}.$$

(a) Show that $\dfrac{\mathrm{d}y}{\mathrm{d}x} = \dfrac{t-1}{t+1}$. **(3 marks)**

(b) Show that the line $x + 3y = 28$ is the normal to the curve at the point where $t = -2$.

**(4 marks)**

(c) Find the value of $t$ at the point where this normal meets the curve again. **(4 marks)**

13. A closed container is made of thin metal in the shape of a cylinder with a hemispherical cap on one end. The radius of the cylinder and cap is $r$ cm and the container is designed to hold $100 \, \text{cm}^3$ precisely.

(a) Show that the area of metal required to make the cap, $A \, \text{cm}^2$, is given by

$$A = \frac{5}{3}\pi r^2 + \frac{200}{r}.$$

**(5 marks)**

(b) Given that $r$ varies, find the minimum volume of $A$ and the volume of $r$ for which it occurs.

Give your answers to 4 significant figures. **(7 marks)**

14. (a) By using integration by parts, show that

$$\int x^2 \sin x \, \mathrm{d}x = 2 \int x \cos x \, \mathrm{d}x - x^2 \cos x.$$

**(4 marks)**

(b) Using a further application of integration by parts, hence find

$$\int x^2 \sin x \, \mathrm{d}x.$$

**(4 marks)**

(c) The finite region $R$ is bounded by the lines $x = \dfrac{\pi}{4}$, $x = \dfrac{\pi}{3}$ and $y = 0$ and the curve with equation $y = x \sin^{\frac{1}{2}} x$. The region $R$ is rotated through $2\pi$ radians about the $x$-axis to form a solid $S$.

Find, to 3 significant figures, the volume of $S$. **(5 marks)**

**Total: 100 marks**

## Longman Examination Board

### General Certificate of Education

### Pure Mathematics and Statistics

### Paper 2 (Pure Mathematics)

**Time: 2 hours**

**Instructions**

■ Answer all questions.

■ Make sure your method is clear, with sufficient working to show how the answer has been obtained.

| Number | Mark |
|--------|------|
| 1. | |
| 2. | |
| 3. | |
| 4. | |
| 5. | |
| 6. | |
| 7. | |
| 8. | |
| 9. | |
| 10. | |
| 11. | |
| 12. | |
| 13. | |
| **Total:** | |

**Information for candidates**

■ The number of marks is given in brackets at the end of each question or part-question.

■ This paper has 13 questions. The maximum mark for this paper is 100.

---

1. Given that $\ln 2 = p$, $\ln 3 = q$, express in terms of $p$ and $q$

   (a) $\ln 6$, **(1 mark)**

   (b) $\ln \frac{3}{4}$, **(1 mark)**

   (c) $\ln\left(\frac{9e}{8}\right)$. **(2 marks)**

2. Obtain and simplify in ascending powers of $x$ the first four terms in the expansion of $(1 - 5x)^8$. **(4 marks)**

3. An inextensible string $AB$ of length $20\,\text{cm}$ is held taut on the outer surface of a cylinder of radius $8\,\text{cm}$ so that it lies in the shape of an arc of a circle. The plane containing the string is at right-angles to the axis of the cylinder.

   Find the length, to the nearest mm, of the straight line joining $A$ to $B$. **(5 marks)**

4. The points $W$, $X$ and $Y$ are at $(4,4)$, $(9,-1)$ and $(2,-2)$ respectively.

   (a) Show that $WX = XY$. **(2 marks)**

   (b) Find the coordinates of the point $Z$ which is the reflection of the point $X$ in the line $WY$. **(3 marks)**

5. Solve the equation $3\cos^2 x = 8\sin x$, giving the values of $x$ in degrees to 1 decimal place which lie in the interval $[0,360°]$. **(5 marks)**

**6.** The $n$th term of a sequence is $u_n$, where

$$u_n = 2 + \frac{2}{u_{n-1} + 1}, \qquad u_1 = 1, \qquad n \geqslant 1.$$

(a) Find the exact values of $u_3$ and $u_4$. **(2 marks)**

The limiting value $x$ of the sequence is found by putting $u_{n-1} = u_n = x$.

(b) Find the value of $x$, giving your answer as a surd. **(4 marks)**

**7.** A curve $C$ has the equation $y = -1 + 3x - \dfrac{x^2}{4}$.

At the point $A$ on $C$, the gradient is $-1$.

Find

(a) the coordinates of $A$, **(4 marks)**

(b) an equation of the normal to $C$ at $A$. **(3 marks)**

**8.** A particle $P$ leaves a fixed point $O$ and moves in a straight line. At time $t$ seconds after leaving $O$, $P$ is $x$ metres from $O$, and $x = 6t^2 - t^3$, where $0 \leqslant t \leqslant 6$. Calculate

(a) the greatest displacement of $P$ from $O$, **(4 marks)**

(b) the greatest speed of $P$ in the interval $0 \leqslant t \leqslant 6$. **(4 marks)**

**9.** The first term of a geometric series is $p$ and the second term is $p^2 - p$.

(a) Find the third term in terms of $p$. **(3 marks)**

(b) Given that $p = \frac{5}{3}$, find

(i) the sum of the first 15 terms, giving your answer to 3 significant figures,
**(4 marks)**

(ii) the exact sum to infinity of the series. **(2 marks)**

**10.** (a) Solve the equation

$$2(x - 3)(x + 1) - (x - 3)^2 = 4x + 13,$$

giving your answers to 2 decimal places. **(6 marks)**

(b) Find the set of values of $x$ for which

$$2(x - 3)(x + 1) > (x - 3)^2$$ **(5 marks)**

**11.** The depreciation in the value of a second-hand car is modelled by assuming that the rate of change in the value, $x$, in pounds, at any time $t$, in months, after the car is bought is proportional to $x$. The car was bought for £5000 when $t = 0$.

(a) Show that $V = 5000e^{-kt}$, where $k$ is a positive constant. **(4 marks)**

(b) After 24 months, the car's value is £3000.

(i) Find the value of the car after 36 months. **(4 marks)**

(ii) Find how long to the nearest month, before the car is worth just £1000.
**(3 marks)**

**Turn over**

**12.** The curve with equation $y = 2\cos x + 1$ is partly shown in the diagram, where the curve meets the $y$-axis at $A$ and the $x$-axis at $B$.

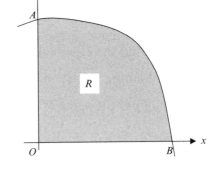

(a) Find the coordinates of $A$ and $B$. **(3 marks)**

(b) The shaded region $R$ is bounded by $OA$, $OB$ and part of the curve, as shown. Using integration, find

(i) the area of $R$, **(4 marks)**

(ii) the volume generated when $R$ is rotated completely about $Ox$. **(5 marks)**

**13.** $$f(x) = \ln x - 8\tan x.$$

(a) Show that the equation $f(x) = 0$ has a root $\alpha$ in the interval $[6.50, 6.52]$. **(2 marks)**

(b) Use linear interpolation on the interval $[6.50, 6.52]$ to estimate $\alpha$, giving your answer to 4 decimal places. **(4 marks)**

(c) Use the Newton–Raphson process on $f(x)$ with 6.50 as a first approximation to $\alpha$ to obtain a second approximation, giving your answer to 4 decimal places. **(5 marks)**

(d) Investigate which of your two answers does in fact give $\alpha$ *correct* to 4 decimal places. **(2 marks)**

**Total: 100 marks**

# Longman
## Examination Board

**General Certificate of Education**

**Pure Mathematics and Statistics**

**Paper 3 (Pure Mathematics)**

**Time: 2 hours**

**Instructions**

- Answer all questions.

- Make sure your method is clear, with sufficient working to show how the answer has been obtained.

| Number | Mark |
|--------|------|
| 1. | |
| 2. | |
| 3. | |
| 4. | |
| 5. | |
| 6. | |
| 7. | |
| 8. | |
| 9. | |
| 10. | |
| 11. | |
| 12. | |
| 13. | |
| **Total:** | |

**Information for candidates**

- The number of marks is given in brackets at the end of each question or part-question.

- This paper has 13 questions. The maximum mark for this paper is 100.

---

1. Given that $180° < x < 270°$, find $x$ if $\sqrt{3} \tan(90° - x) = 1$. **(3 marks)**

2. The function $f(x) = 2x^3 + (3 - 2k)x^2 - x(3k + 2) + 6$, where $k$ is a constant, has a factor $(x - 3)$.

   (a) Find the value of $k$. **(2 marks)**

   (b) Factorise $f(x)$ completely. **(3 marks)**

3. An arithmetic series has first term 23 and common difference 0.2.

   (a) Find the 1000th term in the series. **(2 marks)**

   (b) Find the sum of the first 240 terms in the series. **(3 marks)**

4. Find the set of values of $x$ for which

$$\frac{x^2 + 12}{x} > 7$$ **(6 marks)**

5. The equations of two circles are

$$x^2 + y^2 + 2x + 4y - 20 = 0,$$
$$x^2 + y^2 + 6x - 8y + 24 = 0.$$

**Turn over**

(a) Calculate

    (i)   the radii of the two circles,         **(3 marks)**

    (ii)   the distance between the centres of the two circles.         **(2 marks)**

(b) Deduce that the two circles do not intersect.         **(1 mark)**

**6.** The tangent at the point (2,4) on the curve with equation $y = 8x - 3x^2$ has equation $y = mx + c$.

(a) Find the value of $m$ and of $c$.         **(3 marks)**

    The normal at the point (2,4) to the curve $y = 8x - 3x^2$ meets the $x$-axis and $y$-axis at $A$ and $B$ respectively.

(b) Find the area of triangle $OAB$ where $O$ is the origin.         **(3 marks)**

**7.** The diagram below shows the curve $y = f(x)$ having a stationary point at $(1,-4)$ and cutting the axes at the points $(-1,0)$, $(3,0)$ and $(0,-3)$.

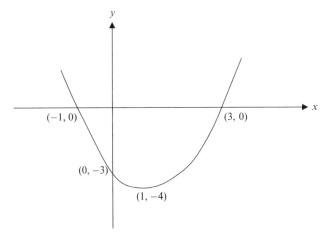

Sketch on separate diagrams the curves

(a)   $y = f(x + 1)$,         **(2 marks)**

(b)   $y = -2f(x)$,         **(2 marks)**

(c)   $y = |f(x)|$.         **(2 marks)**

indicating clearly on each diagram the coordinates of the points where the curves cross the coordinate axes.

**8.** The table below shows corresponding values of the variables $x$ and $y$ obtained in an experiment.

| $x$ | 5 | 10 | 15 | 20 | 25 |
|---|---|---|---|---|---|
| $y$ | 149 | 175 | 219 | 280 | 359 |

(a) By plotting a graph of $y$ against $x^2$ show that these values may be regarded as approximations to values satisfying a relation of the form $y = a + bx^2$ where $a$ and $b$ are constants.         **(2 marks)**

(b) Use your graph to estimate the values of $a$ and $b$ giving your answers to 2 significant figures.         **(4 marks)**

(c) Estimate to 1 decimal place the value of $x$ for which $y = 200$.         **(1 mark)**

**9.** Find the coordinates of the stationary points on the curve with equation $y = \dfrac{x^2}{1 + x^4}$.

        **(8 marks)**

**10.** (a) Using $\cos 2\theta = 1 - 2\sin^2\theta$, find $\int \sin^2\theta\,\mathrm{d}\theta$. **(2 marks)**

(b) The curve with equation $y = 4\sin x$ from $x = 0$ to $x = \pi$ cuts off a finite region $A$ with the $x$-axis as shown in the diagram below.

   (i) Find the area of $A$. **(3 marks)**

   (ii) Find the volume of the solid generated when $A$ is rotated completely about the $x$-axis.

   **(3 marks)**

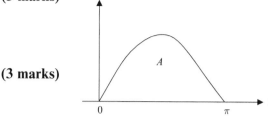

**11.** In the diagram below, the sector $S$ of the circle radius $R$ shown subtends an angle $\phi$ at the centre of the circle. It is rolled up to form the curved surface of a right circular cone standing on a base of radius $r$. The semivertical angle of the cone is $\theta$ radians.

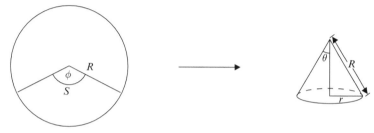

(a) Show that

   (i) $r = R\sin\theta$, **(1 mark)**

   (ii) $\phi = 2\pi\sin\theta$. **(2 marks)**

(b) Show that the volume of the cone is given by $3V = \pi R^3 \sin^2\theta\cos\theta$. **(2 marks)**

(c) Given that $R$ is constant, but $\theta$ is variable, find $\dfrac{\mathrm{d}V}{\mathrm{d}\theta}$ and show that when $\dfrac{\mathrm{d}V}{\mathrm{d}\theta} = 0$, $\tan\theta = \sqrt{2}$ and that the volume of the cone is exactly $\dfrac{2\pi R^3\sqrt{3}}{27}$. **(6 marks)**

(d) Find also the area of the sector $S$ in terms of $R$ in this case. **(2 marks)**

**12.** (a) Using the identity $\cos 3\theta \equiv \cos(2\theta + \theta)$, show that

$$\cos 3\theta = 4\cos^3\theta - 3\cos\theta.$$ **(4 marks)**

(b) Given that $2\cos\theta = x + \dfrac{1}{x}$, show that $2\cos 3\theta = x^3 + \dfrac{1}{x^3}$. **(3 marks)**

(c) Given that when $A$ is small $\cos A \approx 1 - \dfrac{A^2}{2!} + \dfrac{A^4}{4!}$, express $\cos 3\theta$ and $\cos\theta$ in terms of powers of $\theta$ up to and including the term in $\theta^4$.

Hence show that $\cos^3\theta \approx 1 - \dfrac{3\theta^2}{2} + \dfrac{7\theta^4}{8}$. **(3 marks)**

(d) Calculate the relative error in using $\cos^3\theta = 1 - \dfrac{3\theta^2}{2} + \dfrac{7\theta^4}{8}$ as an approximation when $\theta = \dfrac{\pi}{10}$ giving your answer correct to 3 decimal places. **(3 marks)**

**13.** (a) Given $x^3 + 2y^3 + 3xy = 0$, find the value of $\dfrac{\mathrm{d}y}{\mathrm{d}x}$ when $x = 2$ and $y = -1$. **(6 marks)**

(b) Given that $x = e^{2t}\cos 2t$, $y = e^{2t}\sin 2t$, show that

$$\frac{\mathrm{d}y}{\mathrm{d}x} = \tan\left(\frac{\pi}{4} + 2t\right).$$ **(8 marks)**

**Total: 100 marks**

# Longman
# Examination Board

## General Certificate of Education

## Pure Mathematics and Statistics

## Paper 4 (Pure Mathematics)

**Time: 2 hours**

### Instructions

- Answer all questions.

- Make sure your method is clear, with sufficient working to show how the answer has been obtained.

| Number | Mark |
|--------|------|
| 1. | |
| 2. | |
| 3. | |
| 4. | |
| 5. | |
| 6. | |
| 7. | |
| 8. | |
| 9. | |
| 10. | |
| 11. | |
| 12. | |
| **Total:** | |

### Information for candidates

- The number of marks is given in brackets at the end of each question or part-question.

- This paper has 12 questions. The maximum mark for this paper is 100.

---

1. A rectangular field has an area of $75\,940\,\text{m}^2$ (correct to $10\,\text{m}^2$) and a breadth of 101 m (correct to the nearest metre).

   Find the greatest possible length of the field, giving your answer to the nearest metre.

   **(4 marks)**

2. Find the value of $x$ in the interval $(0,360°)$ for which $\sin(2x - 30°) = \sin(x - 40°)$.

   **(4 marks)**

3. A geometric series has first term $a$ and common ratio $r$ where $|r| < 1$. The sum to infinity of the series is 8. When only the odd terms of the series are considered, that is, $a + ar^2 + ar^4 + \cdots$ the sum to infinity of the new series is 6.

   Find the value of $a$ and the value of $r$.

   **(5 marks)**

4. The roots of the equation $x^2 + px + q = 0$ are $a$ and $a + 1$. By comparing the equation with the equation $(x - a)(x - a - 1) = 0$ show that $p^2 = 4q + 1$.  **(5 marks)**

5. The diagram below shows two points, $A$ and $B$, distance 89 m apart on one side of a canal with parallel banks. The point $C$ lies on the opposite bank and $A$, $B$ and $C$ all line in the same horizontal plane, $\angle CAB = 45.6°$, $\angle CBA = 63.1°$.

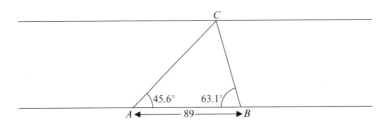

    (a)   Use the sine rule to find the distance of $A$ from $C$. **(4 marks)**

    (b)   Find the width of the canal. **(2 marks)**

**6.**   The sketch below shows the graph of

$$y = |x^2 + 2x - 3|.$$

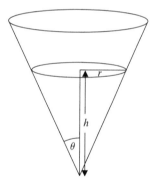

Calculate all four roots of the equation

$$|x^2 + 2x - 3| = 2,$$

expressing your answers in surd form.

Hence solve the inequality $|x^2 + 2x - 3| \leqslant 2$. **(7 marks)**

**7.**   (a)   Expand $(x + 2y)^6$ by the binomial theorem in ascending powers of $y$ up to and including the term in $y^4$. **(3 marks)**

    (b)   Choosing suitable values of $x$ and $y$, evaluate $1.02^6$ correct to 4 decimal places. **(4 marks)**

**8.**   The diagram below shows a hollow inverted right circular cone of semivertical angle $\theta$. It contains a volume $V \, \text{cm}^3$ of water to a height $h \, \text{cm}$ and base radius $r \, \text{cm}$ as shown.

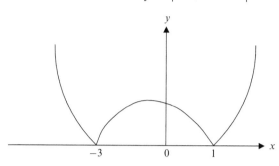

    (a)   Show the area $A \, \text{cm}^2$ of the circular surface of the water is given by $A = \pi h^2 \tan^2 \theta$. **(1 mark)**

    (b)   Show the volume of water $V = \frac{1}{3} \pi h^3 \tan^2 \theta$. **(1 mark)**

    (c)   Water is poured into the container at the rate of $k \, \text{cm}^3 \, \text{s}^{-1}$. Show that the height $h \, \text{cm}$ of the water is increasing at the rate $\dfrac{k}{\pi r^2} \, \text{cm} \, \text{s}^{-1}$. **(4 marks)**

    (d)   Find the rate at which the area $A$ of the circular surface of water is increasing, expressing your answer in terms of $h$ and $k$. **(3 marks)**

**9.**   A curve $C$ has parametric equations

$$x = 4t - \ln 2t, \qquad y = t^2 - \ln t^2, \qquad t > 0$$

    (a)   Find $\dfrac{\mathrm{d}y}{\mathrm{d}x}$ in terms of $t$. **(5 marks)**

**Turn over**

(b) Find the value of $t$ at the point $A$ on the curve at which the gradient is $\frac{1}{2}$. **(3 marks)**

(c) Find, in its simplest form, an equation of the tangent to the curve $C$ at the point $A$.
**(4 marks)**

10. (a) Express $\dfrac{x^2 + 2x - 4}{(x + 1)(x^2 + 4)}$ in the form $\dfrac{A}{x + 1} + \dfrac{Bx + C}{x^2 + 4}$.

Hence evaluate $\displaystyle\int_1^4 \dfrac{x^2 + 2x - 4}{(x + 1)(x^2 + 4)}\,\mathrm{d}x$ leaving your answer in the form $\ln\left(\dfrac{P}{Q}\right)$ where $P$ and $Q$ are numbers to be found. **(7 marks)**

(b) Use integration by parts to find $\displaystyle\int \ln x\,\mathrm{d}x$. Hence or otherwise find the general solution of the differential equation $\dfrac{\mathrm{d}y}{\mathrm{d}x} = \sec 2y \cdot \ln x$. **(6 marks)**

11. The function f is defined by f: $x \mapsto x^2 - 9$, $x \in \mathbb{R}$, $x > 0$.

(a) Sketch the graph of f showing on your sketch the coordinates of any points where the curve meets the axes. **(2 marks)**

(b) Find, in the same form as f, the inverse function $f^{-1}$ and state (i) its domain, and (ii) its range. **(5 marks)**

(c) Sketch the graph of $f^{-1}$ on the same axes as you used for (a), distinguishing clearly between f and $f^{-1}$. **(2 marks)**

(d) Find the value of $x$ for which $f(x) = 4x$, giving your answer in surd form. **(2 marks)**

(e) Show clearly why the $x$-coordinate of the point of intersection of the curves $y = f(x)$ and $y = f^{-1}(x)$ is given by one root of the equation $x^2 - x - 9 = 0$. Find the root giving your answer to 3 significant figures. **(3 marks)**

12. The diagram below shows the intersection of the curve $y = \dfrac{6}{x}$ and the straight line $y = 9 - 3x$.

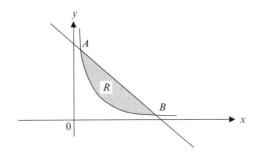

(a) Find the coordinates of the points of intersection $A$ and $B$. **(4 marks)**

(b) Find the area of the shaded region $R$. **(5 marks)**

(c) Find the volume obtained when the shaded region $R$ is revolved completely about the $x$-axis. **(5 marks)**

**Total: 100 marks**

# Longman
# Examination Board

## General Certificate of Education

## Pure Mathematics and Statistics

## Paper 5 (Statistics)

**Time: 2 hours**

| Number | Mark |
|--------|------|
| 1. | |
| 2. | |
| 3. | |
| 4. | |
| 5. | |
| 6. | |
| 7. | |
| 8. | |
| 9. | |
| 10. | |
| 11. | |
| **Total:** | |

### Instructions

- Answer all questions.

- Make sure your method is clear, with sufficient working to show how the answer has been obtained.

### Information for candidates

- The number of marks is given in brackets at the end of each question or part-question.

- This paper has 11 questions. The maximum mark for this paper is 100.

---

1. Explain briefly the use of

   (a)   (i)   a census, **(1 mark)**

         (ii)   a sample survey. **(1 mark)**

   (b)   Give an example of each. **(2 marks)**

2. The following scores were recorded by a golfer playing a four-hole approach and putt course:

   $$13, 17, 21, 22, 19, 17, 17, 16, 16, 12, 20, 20, 18, 17, 21, 15, 19, 17, 16, 21$$

   Calculate

   (a)   his mean score, **(2 marks)**

   (b)   the standard deviation of his scores. **(3 marks)**

3. Boxes $A$ and $B$ contain a number of red, white and blue balls, all of equal size, as shown in the table below.

   | | **Red** | **White** | **Blue** |
   |-------|-----|-------|------|
   | **Box $A$** | 3 | 2 | 1 |
   | **Box $B$** | 0 | 4 | 2 |

   The balls in box $A$ have twice the chance of being drawn as those in box $B$.

   A ball is drawn from a box. Find the probability that

   (a)   a white ball is drawn, **(3 marks)**

   (b)   box $A$ was used, given that a white ball is drawn. **(4 marks)**

   **Turn over**

4. There are about 50 000 members in a professional association of civil servants. From a random sample of 120 members, the mean age was 47.5 years and the standard deviation was 19.3 years. Determine a 95% confidence interval for the mean age of all the members of the association. **(7 marks)**

5. A car dealer has two branches, *A* and *B*, in the same city and they each have an independnet switchboard for receiving phone calls. During the period from 1230 to 1430 it has been observed over a long time that the number of calls received at *A* had a Poisson distribution with parameter 4, while the independent number received at *B* has a Poisson distribution with parameter 5. Giving answers to 2 significant figures, estimate the probability for a day chosen at random that, from 1230 to 1430

   (a) there are precisely 5 calls to *A*, **(2 marks)**

   (b) there are at least 3 calls to *B*, **(3 marks)**

   (c) there are exactly 3 calls to *A* and *B* together. **(3 marks)**

6. In a survey, 1000 randomly chosen women from a district were asked whether they would buy a new product and 357 replied YES.

   (a) Find a 95% confidence interval for the proportion *p* of the whole population of women who would answer YES to the same question. **(6 marks)**

   (b) In all, 20 similar surveys (including this one) were conducted nationwide and the 95% confidence interval was found for each survey. State the expected number of these which would enclose the true value of *p*. **(2 marks)**

7. The table below shows the rankings given to 10 entries in a Dahlia Growing Competition at a local flower show.

| | A | B | C | D | E | F | G | H | I | J |
|---|---|---|---|---|---|---|---|---|---|---|
| **Rank (1st Judge)** | 1 | 2 | 3 | 4 | 5 | 6 | 7 | 8 | 9 | 10 |
| **Rank (2nd Judge)** | 2 | 6 | 4 | 3 | 1 | 7 | 5 | 10 | 8 | 9 |

   (a) Calculate Spearman's Coefficient of Rank Correlation between the rankings of the two judges. **(5 marks)**

   (b) Using a table of critical values, comment on the significance of the value at the 5% level and at the 1% level, stating the null hypothesis in each case. **(5 marks)**

8. The discrete random variable *X* has probability function

$$P(X = x) = \begin{cases} kx & \text{for } x = 1, 3, 5, 7, 9 \\ 0 & \text{otherwise.} \end{cases}$$

   Find the value of

   (a) *k*, **(2 marks)**

   (b) $E(X)$, **(3 marks)**

   (c) $\text{Var}(X)$, **(3 marks)**

   (d) $\text{Var}(2x - 4)$. **(3 marks)**

9. (a) State two assumptions which you should always make when applying a binomial distribution analysis to a statistical problem. **(2 marks)**

(b)  A market gardener sows sweet-pea seeds 12 in a box, and the probability of any seed germinating is 0.9. For a box chosen at random, find, giving answers to 3 significant figures, the probability that

   (i)  all 12 seeds germinate, **(2 marks)**

   (ii)  exactly 10 of the seeds germinate, **(3 marks)**

   (iii)  at least 10 of the seeds germinate. **(4 marks)**

10. The weight of soap powder in a randomly selected packet is normally distributed with a mean of 625 g and a standard deviation of 15 g. The weight of the packet containing soap powder is independent of the contents and is normally distributed with a mean of 25 g and a standard deviation of 3 g. Estimate the probability that

(a)  a randomly chosen packet of soap powder has a total weight exceeding 630 g, **(6 marks)**

(b)  the total weight of the *contents* of 4 randomly selected packets exceeds 2450 g. **(6 marks)**

11. The continuous random variable $X$ has probability density function f, given by

$$f(x) = \begin{cases} c & \text{if } 0 \leqslant x \leqslant 2, \\ c(3-x) & \text{if } 2 < x \leqslant 3, \\ 0 & \text{otherwise,} \end{cases} \quad c \text{ is a constant}$$

(a)  Sketch the graph of f. **(2 marks)**

(b)  Show that $c = 0.4$. **(2 marks)**

(c)  Evaluate $E(X)$ and find the median of $X$. **(8 marks)**

(d)  Find the variance of $X$. **(5 marks)**

**Total: 100 marks**

# Longman Examination Board

## General Certificate of Education

## Pure Mathematics and Statistics

## Paper 6 (Statistics)

**Time: 2 hours**

| Number | Mark |
|--------|------|
| 1. | |
| 2. | |
| 3. | |
| 4. | |
| 5. | |
| 6. | |
| 7. | |
| 8. | |
| 9. | |
| 10. | |
| **Total:** | |

**Instructions**

■ Answer all questions.

■ Make sure your method is clear, with sufficient working to show how the answer has been obtained.

**Information for candidates**

■ The number of marks is given in brackets at the end of each question or part-question.

■ This paper has 10 questions. The maximum mark for this paper is 100.

---

1. (a) State the conditions under which a binomial distribution may be used as a model for a variate. **(3 marks)**

   (b) For each of the variates described below, state whether or not a binomial distribution is a suitable model. If it is, state the value of $n$ and the probability $p$.

   (i) The number of sixes obtained in 10 consecutive throws of a die.

   (ii) The number of times a card must be dealt from a well shuffled pack before an ace is obtained.

   (iii) The number of children in a school of 500 pupils whose birthday falls on a Sunday during the 28 days of February. **(5 marks)**

2. Thirty children in a class were asked to record the number of hours $x$ they each spent reading during their two-week Easter holiday. On return to school after the holiday it was found that $\sum x = 315$ and $\sum x^2 = 3350$.

   (a) If $\mu$ and $\sigma$ are the mean and standard deviation, respectively, of the number of hours spent reading by the children during the holiday, calculate

   (i) $\mu$, **(2 marks)**

   (ii) $\sigma$. **(2 marks)**

   (b) Two extra children who were absent from the school just before the holiday began, claim to have read for 9 hours and 12 hours during the two weeks. If their reading times had been included in the calculations, decide, giving reasons for your decisions, whether they would have affected the values for

   (i) the mean $\mu$, **(2 marks)**

   (ii) the standard deviation. **(2 marks)**

3.  After a number of accidents at a busy road junction, the residents in the neighbourhood called a meeting to discuss asking for the installation of traffic lights. Of the 100 people attending the meeting, 14 of the 34 men and 41 of the 66 women favoured calling for the installation of traffic lights.

    Calculate an approximate symmetric 95% confidence interval for the difference between the proportions of men and women living in the neighbourhood who support the idea of calling for the installation of traffic lights. **(8 marks)**

4.  The heights of girls in a particular year group in a school are normally distributed. Given that 10% of the girls have height greater than 153.2 cm and 20% have height less than 138.6 cm, find

    (a)  the mean height of the girls in the group, **(5 marks)**

    (b)  the standard deviation of their heights. **(3 marks)**

5.  The length of the inside of pencil boxes is a random variable $X \sim N(19, 0.02)$. The length of the pencils to go in the box is a random variable $Y \sim N(18.6, 0.01)$.

    What percentage of pencils will not fit in a randomly chosen box? **(9 marks)**

6.  In a game of chance a person throws two unbiased dice. Each die has 3 red faces, 2 blue faces and 1 gold face.

    For each gold face showing the thrower receives £1.80 from the bank.

    For each red face showing the thrower receives 6p from the bank.

    For each blue face showing the thrower must pay the bank 72p.

    Given that it costs 20p to play the game, find the thrower's expectation. **(10 marks)**

7.  The order in which 15 boys came in a Pure Mathematics examination and a Statistics examination is shown in the table below.

| | A | B | C | D | E | F | G | H | I | J | K | L | M | N | O |
|---|---|---|---|---|---|---|---|---|---|---|---|---|---|---|---|
| **Pure Mathematics** | 1 | 5 | 11 | 8 | 12 | 9 | 2 | 13 | 3 | 15 | 7 | 4 | 10 | 14 | 6 |
| **Statistics** | 3 | 9 | 14 | 11 | 15 | 6 | 2 | 12 | 1 | 10 | 5 | 7 | 13 | 8 | 4 |

    (a)  Calculate Spearman's rank correlation coefficient. **(5 marks)**

    (b)  Use a suitable test at the 5% significance level to investigate the assertion that there is no correlation between the two sets of results, stating clearly the null and alternative hypotheses used. **(5 marks)**

8.  A soft fruit firm concerned with the number of hours that strawberries may be kept after picking before being sent to market is asked to consider using the random variable $X$ (in units of 8 hours) along with the probability density function f given by

$$f(x) = K - \frac{1}{16}x^2 \qquad 0 \leqslant x \leqslant 4, \qquad K \text{ a constant}$$
$$= 0 \qquad\qquad \text{otherwise}$$

    (a)  Find the value of $K$. **(3 marks)**

    (b)  Find the mean number of hours the strawberries may be kept. **(4 marks)**

    (c)  Find the probability that the delay in sending them to market is greater than 8 hours. **(3 marks)**

    **Turn over**

(d) The strawberries could be subjected to radiation treatment and then the delay in sending them to market could be 35 hours. Explain why the same random variable $X$ with probability function f as above would not be a suitable model in this case.

**(2 marks)**

9. In the manufacture of woollen blankets of size 220 cm by 190 cm, small faults occur at random in the weaving. It is found that the average number of faults per blanket is 2.5. Given that the number of faults follows a Poisson distribution,

(a) calculate the probability that a blanket chosen at random will be free of faults.

**(2 marks)**

(b) Find the probability that 3 blankets chosen at random will have a total of no more than 4 faults. **(6 marks)**

(c) A second batch of material is used and it is found that blankets chosen at random now have an average of 15 faults per blanket. Using a suitable approximation find the probability that a randomly selected blanket contains fewer than 9 faults. **(5 marks)**

10. The marks obtained by 51 students in a class taking a Statistics examination paper are given below.

$$
\begin{array}{cccccc}
47 & 28 & 75 & 42 & 37 & 80 \\
71 & 48 & 66 & 41 & 73 & 37 \\
58 & 30 & 45 & 36 & 27 & 57 \\
45 & 60 & 35 & 72 & 45 & 43 \\
74 & 61 & 38 & 44 & 46 & 52 \\
29 & 54 & 35 & 24 & 61 & 56 \\
54 & 77 & 82 & 44 & 65 & 21 \\
34 & 43 & 23 & 84 & 32 & 63 \\
51 & 74 & 48 & & &
\end{array}
$$

(a) Construct an ordered stem and leaf diagram to represent these data and determine the values of the quartiles and the mean value. **(8 marks)**

(b) Construct a box and whiskers plot and comment on the skewness of the distribution.

**(3 marks)**

(c) State the mode of the distribution and the semi-interquartile range. **(3 marks)**

**Total: 100 marks**

## Longman
## Examination Board

**General Certificate of Education**

**Pure Mathematics and Statistics**

**Paper 7 (Statistics)**

**Time: 2 hours**

**Instructions**

■  Answer all questions.

■  Make sure your method is clear, with sufficient working to show how the answer has been obtained.

| Number | Mark |
|--------|------|
| 1. | |
| 2. | |
| 3. | |
| 4. | |
| 5. | |
| 6. | |
| 7. | |
| 8. | |
| 9. | |
| Total: | |

**Information for candidates**

■  The number of marks is given in brackets at the end of each question or part-question.

■  This paper has 9 questions. The maximum mark for this paper is 100.

---

1.  In hypothesis testing, state the type of error that may be made in each of the following cases.

    (a)  The conclusion is to reject the null hypothesis.                    **(1 mark)**

    (b)  The conclusion is to fail to reject the null hypothesis.            **(1 mark)**

    (c)  The calculated value of the test statistic lies outside the critical region.    **(1 mark)**

2.  The weight $w$ kg of each girl in a random sample of 150 teenage girls living in London was measured. Their total weight was found to be $\sum_{r=1}^{150} w_r = 7545$ with $\sum_{r=1}^{150} w_r^2 = 381106$.

    (a)  Calculate unbiased estimates of the mean and variance of this random sample of teenage girls.                                                              **(4 marks)**

    (b)  Determine an approximate 95% confidence interval of the mean weight of teenage girls living in London.                                                       **(3 marks)**

3.  A company doctor is of the opinion that increased stress leads to increased blood pressure. The doctor therefore decides to consider the relationship between the age $x$ years and the systolic blood pressure $y$ millimetres of mercury of 10 randomly chosen women in the firm whom the doctor believes to be vulnerable to stress. The results are given in the table below.

| Age $x$ | 36.2 | 38.5 | 42.0 | 42.3 | 47.2 | 47.6 | 49.6 | 52.3 | 54.3 | 56.1 |
|---------|------|------|------|------|------|------|------|------|------|------|
| Blood pressure $y$ | 118 | 135 | 144 | 139 | 145 | 151 | 153 | 160 | 158 | 161 |

$\sum x = 466.1$     $\sum y = 1464$     $\sum xy = 68996.7$     $\sum x^2 = 22130.73$

**Turn over**

(a) Plot a scatter diagram of the data. **(3 marks)**

(b) Calculate the least square regression equation of $y$ on $x$ and show the line on your scatter diagram. **(6 marks)**

(c) Given that blood pressure of women in this age range should not really exceed $(100 + \text{age})$ mm of mercury, draw a line to represent this upper limit on your graph. Comment with reasons based on this evidence whether you think the doctor's opinion has substance. **(2 marks)**

4. A multiple choice examination paper requires a candidate to answer 100 questions. Each question has 3 answers, only one of which is correct. The pass mark is 40 correct answers. The candidate decides to answer all of the questions randomly.

(a) Use the normal distribution as an approximation to the binomial distribution to estimate the probability that the candidate will pass the examination. **(5 marks)**

(b) The number of questions on the paper is reduced, but the pass mark remains 40 correct answers.

If the candidate is now to have a chance of no more than 5% of passing the examination, still answering the questions randomly, what is the maximum number of questions the paper should contain? **(6 marks)**

5. The number of times a lift in an office block broke down each week was recorded over a two-year period, with the following results.

| Number of breakdowns each week | 0 | 1 | 2 | 3 | 4 | 5 |
|---|---|---|---|---|---|---|
| Frequency | 23 | 25 | 25 | 17 | 9 | 5 |

It is believed that the figure may be modelled by a Poisson distribution.

(a) Give reasons why this may be so. **(2 marks)**

(b) Calculate, correct to 2 significant figures, an estimate of the possible mean $\lambda$. **(1 mark)**

(c) Using your answer to (b), construct a test at the 0.05 level of significance to see whether such a belief is reasonable. State clearly your null and alternative hypotheses. **(9 marks)**

6. Tickets numbered 1 to 5 are placed in box $A$. Tickets numbered 11–18 are placed in box $B$. Mr Jones is asked to choose at random a ticket from one of the boxes.

(a) Using a tree diagram, find the probability that Mr Jones chose an even-numbered ticket. **(5 marks)**

(b) Given that Mr Jones chose an odd-numbered ticket, find the probability that it was chosen from Box A. **(3 marks)**

(c) Mr Jones was asked to choose two tickets, one after the other without replacement.

Find the probability that Mr Jones chose one odd and one even ticket. **(5 marks)**

7. A drug company has two drugs, $A$ and $B$, to help reduce pain for those suffering from arthritis. The drugs are administered to two groups of patients. Group $G_1$ was treated with drug $A$, and 60 of the 90 patients in group $G_1$ found increased relief. Group $G_2$ was treated with drug $B$, and 50 of the 80 patients in group $G_2$ found increased relief.

(a) Find an approximate 95% confidence interval for the population proportion for which $A$ is effective. State why your interval is approximate. **(5 marks)**

(b) Test at the 10% significance level if there is any difference between the effectiveness of the two drugs. **(8 marks)**

**8.** The Editor of the broadsheet *Daily Recorder* decides to change the paper to tabloid form. He claims that 25% of its readers favour the new format in preference to the old format.

    (a) Assuming this figure to be correct, calculate, using the binomial distribution, the probability that in a random sample of 6 readers, at least 2 of them prefer the new format. **(4 marks)**

    (b) Using a suitable approximation, calculate the probability that in a random sample of 250 readers, between 45 and 70 prefer the new format. **(7 marks)**

    (c) In order to test the Editor's assertion, 200 *Daily Recorder* readers are interviewed and 45 prefer the new format. Test whether this result provides significant evidence at the 5% level that the Editor is correct in claiming as much as 25% support for the new format. **(4 marks)**

**9.** The members of two groups, $A$ and $B$, all have a disease. A serum is given to those in group $A$, but not to those in group $B$. Group $A$ contains 80 people; group $B$ contains 120 people. 65 of those in group $A$ recover from the disease, but only 80 of those in group $B$ recover. Test, using a $2 \times 2$ contingency table, the hypothesis that the serum helps to cure the disease at

    (i) the 5% level of significance,

    (ii) the 2.5% level of significance. **(15 marks)**

**Total: 100 marks**

# Longman Examination Board

## General Certificate of Education

## Pure Mathematics and Statistics

## Paper 8 (Statistics)

**Time: 2 hours**

**Instructions**

■ Answer all questions.

■ Make sure your method is clear, with sufficient working to show how the answer has been obtained.

**Information for candidates**

■ The number of marks is given in brackets at the end of each question or part-question.

■ This paper has 9 questions. The maximum mark for this paper is 100.

| Number | Mark |
|--------|------|
| 1. | |
| 2. | |
| 3. | |
| 4. | |
| 5. | |
| 6. | |
| 7. | |
| 8. | |
| 9. | |
| Total: | |

---

1. A probability distribution of the discrete random variable $X$ is given in the table below.

   | $X$ | 1 | 2 | 3 | 4 |
   |-----|---|---|---|---|
   | $P(X)$ | $K$ | $8K$ | $27K$ | $64K$ |

   Find

   (a) the value of $K$, **(1 mark)**

   (b) the mean and variance of the distribution, **(4 marks)**

   (c) the mean and variance of $4X - 5$. **(3 marks)**

2. Jean and Ann work for a garment manufacturer. Jean is a fully trained machinist and Ann is a trainee machinist. The probability that a dress made by Ann contains 1 or more errors is 0.25, but the probability that a dress made by Jean contains 1 or more errors is 0.05.

   (a) Calculate the probability that, of 4 dresses made by Ann, exactly 1 is free of any errors. **(2 marks)**

   (b) Use the cumulative binomial probability tables to find the probability that, in a random sample of 20 dresses made by Jean, not more than 3 of them will contain errors. **(1 mark)**

   (c) On any one day Ann makes 15% of the total of dresses made by Jean and Ann. One of the dresses made by Jean and Ann on one day is chosen at random. Find the probability that it contains 1 or more errors. **(3 marks)**

   (d) On one particular day two dresses are chosen at random from those known to have errors. Find the probability that Jean and Ann each made one of them. **(4 marks)**

22

3. Six samples of iron ore are analysed in order to obtain figures for the percentage of two elements, $X$ and $Y$, contained within each sample. The results are shown in the table below.

| Samples | 1 | 2 | 3 | 4 | 5 | 6 |
|---|---|---|---|---|---|---|
| Element $X$ | 0.81 | 0.48 | 0.53 | 0.45 | 0.71 | 1.02 |
| Element $Y$ | 1.15 | 0.76 | 0.97 | 0.86 | 1.21 | 1.32 |

(a) Given

$$\sum XY = 4.4029 \qquad \sum X^2 = 2.9144 \quad \text{and} \quad \sum Y^2 = 6.7871$$

find, to 3 decimal places, the product moment correlation coefficient of the percentages of the two elements. **(5 marks)**

(b) Calculate also, to 3 decimal places, the Spearman rank correlation coefficient. **(5 marks)**

4. A flour refinery packs flour in bags which have weights normally distributed with mean 1.5 kg and variance 0.01 kg. A check leads the manager to suspect that there has been a slight drift in the machine so that the weights of the bags are no longer 1.5 kg.

A random sample of 100 bags of flour are reweighted and found to have a mean weight of 1.524 kg.

(a) Stating clearly your null and alternative hypotheses, undertake a significance test at the 1% level to determine whether the overall mean weight of the bags of flour is still 1.5 kg. **(8 marks)**

(b) The manager is really only concerned that the bags of flour are not underweight. What form should the hypotheses take and what conclusions should be reached as a result of the significance test at the 1% level? **(2 marks)**

5. The number of breakdown calls received at an AA office in $t$ minutes over a Bank Holiday weekend is known to follow a Poisson distribution with mean $\dfrac{t}{125}$.

(a) Find the probability that the number of calls received from 9.00 a.m. to 9.15 a.m. is greater than 2. **(4 marks)**

(b) Find, to the nearest minute, the length of time that the phone can be left unmanned for there to be a probability of 0.95 that no emergency calls will be received. **(3 marks)**

(c) During a period of heavy snow the office received 9 emergency calls in the $12\frac{1}{2}$-hour shift. Use probability tables or otherwise to determine whether the increase in the average number of emergency calls is significant at the 5% level. **(4 marks)**

6. A well known soap manufacturing company placed a new washing powder on the market. After a six-month period, the company asked a market research agency to find out how well known the powder had become. The agency took a random sample of 900 people and discovered that 198 of them knew of 'Improved Brand X'. Six months later, after further TV advertising, another random sample of 600 people were interviewed and it was discovered that 150 of them knew of 'Improved Brand X'. In order to know whether there had been an increase in the number of people knowing of 'Improved Brand X', a hypothesis test was undertaken.

(a) State whether it should be a one-tailed test. **(2 marks)**

(b) State your hypotheses and use a 5% level of significance. **(9 marks)**

**Turn over**

7.  A school debated the statement, 'This school believes that fox hunting should be abolished.' At the end of the debating session the boys and girls voted as shown in the table below.

| | For the motion | Against the motion | Undecided |
|---|---|---|---|
| Girls | 98 | 42 | 15 |
| Boys | 65 | 56 | 19 |

Test the hypothesis at the 5% level of significance that there is a difference of opinion between the girls and boys as far as the proposal is concerned. **(13 marks)**

8.  The height in cms of a random sample of 72 Sixth Form students in the county of Yorkshire are given in the table below.

| Height | 150– | 155– | 160– | 165– | 170– | 175– | 180– | 185– | 190– | 195– |
|---|---|---|---|---|---|---|---|---|---|---|
| Frequency | 2 | 5 | 4 | 9 | 20 | 12 | 9 | 7 | 3 | 1 |

(a) Estimate the mean height to 4 significant figures. **(2 marks)**

(b) Estimate the standard deviation of this sample of heights. **(2 marks)**

(c) Draw on graph paper a cumulative frequency polygon for this data. **(2 marks)**

(d) Find the median height $Q_2$ and the first and third quartiles $Q_1$ and $Q_3$. Compare the values of $Q_3 - Q_2$ and $Q_2 - Q_1$ and state what this implies about the distribution. **(4 marks)**

(e) Find unbiased estimates of the mean and variance of all Sixth Formers in Yorkshire. **(3 marks)**

9.  The continuous random variable $X$ has cumulative distribution function $F$ given by

$$F(x) = 0 \quad \text{for } x < 0,$$
$$F(x) = \tfrac{1}{18}ax^2 - \tfrac{1}{27}x^3, \quad 0 \leqslant x \leqslant 3, \quad a \text{ a constant},$$
$$F(x) = 1 \quad \text{for } x > 3.$$

(a) Find the value of $a$. **(2 marks)**

(b) Find the probability density function f of $X$. **(3 marks)**

(c) Determine the modal value of $X$. **(1 mark)**

(d) Show that $m$, the median value of $X$, satisfies the equation $2m^3 - 12m^2 + 27 = 0$ and verify that the value of $m$ lies between 1.79 and 1.8. **(3 marks)**

(e) Find $E(X)$ and $\text{Var}(X)$. **(5 marks)**

**Total: 100 marks**

# Solutions to practice exam papers

An explanation of the marking system is given at the front of the book.

Use the following solutions to mark your papers, then look at the mark analysis on page iv.

## Solutions to Paper I (Pure Mathematics)

1. Reduce both sides to powers of 3 only

$$27(3^x) = 3^3 \times 3^x = 3^{x+3} \quad \textbf{M1}$$

$$9^{3x} = (3^2)^{3x} = 3^{6x} \quad \textbf{A1}$$

Then $6x = x + 3 \implies x = \frac{3}{5}$    **A1**    **3 marks**

> **TIP**
>
> The key here is to get both sides to the same base.

2. Put $y = \dfrac{x-3}{2x-4}$, that is $y(2x-4) = x - 3$

$$2xy - 4y = x - 3$$
$$2xy - x = 4y - 3$$
$$x(2y - 1) = 4y - 3 \quad \textbf{M1}$$
$$x = \frac{4y - 3}{2y - 1} \quad \textbf{A1}$$

Now interchange $x$ and $y$ to give

$$y = \frac{4x - 3}{2x - 1}$$

$$f^{-1}: x \mapsto \frac{4x - 3}{2x - 1}, \quad x \neq \frac{1}{2} \quad \textbf{A1} \quad \textbf{A1} \quad \textbf{4 marks}$$

> **TIP**
>
> Note the steps involved in this standard process. Write $y = f(x)$, process through to get $x$ in terms of $y$; change over $x$ and $y$; then write your answer in the form asked for.

3. First, we solve $x + 2y = 3$, $2x + y = 1$ simultaneously to get $x = -\frac{1}{3}$, $y = \frac{5}{3}$   **M1**   **A1**   **A1**

The point $(-\frac{1}{3}, \frac{5}{3})$ also lies on $\lambda x + 3y = 4$ so we have $\lambda(-\frac{1}{3}) + 3(\frac{5}{3}) = 4$    **M1**

$-\lambda + 15 = 12 \implies \lambda = 3$    **A1**    **5 marks**

> **TIP**
>
> Start by solving $x + 2y = 3$, $2x + y = 1$ to find the point of intersection.

4. $f(x) \equiv 5x^3 + Ax^2 - 8x + 4$

   (a) If $x - 2$ is a factor, then $f(2) = 0$

   $$5(2^3) + A(2^2) - 8(2) + 4 = 0 \quad \textbf{M1}$$

   $$40 + 4A - 16 + 4 = 0 \implies A = -7 \quad \textbf{A1} \quad \textbf{2 marks}$$

   (b) $5x^3 - 7x^2 - 8x + 4 = (x - 2)(5x^2 + 3x - 2)$    **M1**

   $$= (x - 2)(5x - 2)(x + 1) \quad \textbf{M1} \quad \textbf{A1} \quad \textbf{3 marks}$$

**TIP**

In (b) line 1, get to $(x - 2)(5x^2 \cdots - 2)$ first, then you can obtain the middle term by noting that $-7x^2$ on the left has to be obtained on the right from $-10x^2$ and $x$ times your $x$ term in the quadratic; that is, then $+3x$ to give $3x^2$ overall. Now check on the $x$ terms where you have $3x \times -2 + x \times -2 = -8x$, which corresponds with the left-hand side.

**5.** $\dfrac{\mathrm{d}y}{\mathrm{d}x} = y \cot x$

$\dfrac{1}{y} \dfrac{\mathrm{d}y}{\mathrm{d}x} = \dfrac{\cos x}{\sin x}$ or $\displaystyle\int \dfrac{1}{y} \, \mathrm{d}y = \int \dfrac{\cos x}{\sin x} \, \mathrm{d}x$ **M1**

Integrating with respect to $x$ we have

$\ln y = \ln \sin x + \text{Constant}$ **A1** **A1**

$y = 2, x = \dfrac{\pi}{6}$ so $\ln 2 = \ln \frac{1}{2} + \text{Constant}$

$\text{Constant} = 2 \ln 2 = \ln 4$ **M1**

$\ln y = \ln \sin x + \ln 4$

$y = 4 \sin x$ is the solution. **A1** **5 marks**

**TIP**

Separate the variables. Note how to eliminate the logarithms to obtain the simplest form.

**6.** $a = 16$, $ar^{12} = 2$ **M1**

$r^{12} = \dfrac{1}{8} = \dfrac{1}{2^3} \Rightarrow r = 2^{-\frac{1}{4}}$ **M1** **A1**

$S_\infty = \dfrac{a}{1-r} = \dfrac{16}{1 - 2^{-\frac{1}{4}}} = 100.6$ (to 4 significant figures) **M1** **A1** **5 marks**

**TIP**

Find the common ratio $r$.

**7.** $\overrightarrow{OR} = 24\mathbf{i} + 7\mathbf{j}$, $\overrightarrow{OS} = 15\mathbf{i} + 20\mathbf{j}$

(a) $|\overrightarrow{OR}| = \sqrt{(24^2 + 7^2)} = 25$, $|\overrightarrow{OS}| = \sqrt{(15^2 + 20^2)} = 25$ **M1**

$|\overrightarrow{OR}| = |\overrightarrow{OS}|$ **A1** **2 marks**

(b) Using scalar product of $\overrightarrow{OR} \cdot \overrightarrow{OS}$, we have

$\cos \angle ROS = \dfrac{\overrightarrow{OR} \cdot \overrightarrow{OS}}{|\overrightarrow{OR}| \cdot |\overrightarrow{OS}|} = \dfrac{24 \times 15 + 7 \times 20}{25 \times 25}$ **M1**

$\angle ROS = 36.87°$ **A1**

Since $\triangle ROS$ is isoceles $\angle ORS = \dfrac{180° - 36.87°}{2} = 71.6°$ (to 1 decimal place)

**M1** **A1** **4 marks**

**TIP**

Use the isosceles triangle rather than the cosine rule.

**8.** (a) Gradient of $PQ = \dfrac{4-0}{\ln 4 - 3} = -2.48$ (to 3 significant figures)  **M1  A1  2 marks**

(b) Area of shaded region = area under curve + area of $\triangle$  **M1**

$$\int e^x \, dx = e^x \quad \textbf{B1}$$

Area under curve $= [e^x]_0^{\ln 4} = e^{\ln 4} - e^0 = 4 - 1 = 3$  **A1**

Area of $\triangle = \frac{1}{2} \times 4 \times (3 - \ln 4) = 3.227$  **A1**

Area of shaded region $= 6.227$  **A1  5 marks**

> **TIP**
>
> Note that $e^{\ln p} = p$.

**9.** (a) Differentiating with respect to $x$

$$3y^2 \frac{dy}{dx} + 2y^2 + 4xy \frac{dy}{dx} = 0 \quad \textbf{B1  M1  A1}$$

$$\frac{dy}{dx} = \frac{-2y}{3y + 4x} \quad \textbf{A1} \qquad \textbf{4 marks}$$

(b) At $P$, $y = -2$, $x = 3$ and $\dfrac{dy}{dx} = \dfrac{2}{3}$  **B1  M1**

Tangent at $P$ has equation $y + 2 = \frac{2}{3}(x - 3)$  **A1  3 marks**

> **TIP**
>
> Remember
>
> $$\frac{d}{dx}(y^3) = \frac{dy}{dx} \cdot \frac{d}{dy}(y^3).$$

**10.** (a) Curve $y = A \sin x + B \cos x$ passes through $(0, -3)$

$\therefore \quad -3 = A \times 0 + B \times 1 \Rightarrow B = -3$  **B1**

Curve also passes through $\left( \dfrac{\pi}{4}, \sqrt{2} \right)$

$\therefore \quad A \times \dfrac{1}{\sqrt{2}} + B \times \dfrac{1}{\sqrt{2}} = \sqrt{2} \Rightarrow A + B = 2$  **M1  A1**

Hence $A = 5$  **A1  4 marks**

(b) $y = 0 \Rightarrow 5 \sin x - 3 \cos x = 0$  **M1**

$\tan x = \dfrac{3}{5}$  **A1**

$x = 0.54$  or  $3.68$  **A1  A1  4 marks**

> **TIP**
>
> Remember $\tan \alpha = \tan(x + \pi)$.

**11.** (a) Acceleration $= \dfrac{dv}{dt} = 4t - 3$  **M1**

$t = 4$, acceleration $= 13 \, \text{ms}^{-2}$  **A1  2 marks**

(b)  Distance $= \int (2t^2 - 3t + 4)\,dt = \left[ \frac{2}{3}t^3 - \frac{3t^2}{2} + 4t \right]$   **M1  A1**

Using limits $1\frac{1}{2}$ to 3 $\Rightarrow$ distance $= \frac{2}{3}(3^3 - 1\frac{1}{2}^3) - \frac{3}{2}(3^2 - 1\frac{1}{2}^2) + 12 - 6$   **M1**

Distance $= 11.625$ metres or $11\frac{5}{8}$ metres.   **A1    4 marks**

(c)  Minimum speed occurs when acceleration $= 0$, that is $t = \frac{3}{4}$   **M1**

Minimum $V = 2(\frac{3}{4})^2 - 3(\frac{3}{4}) + 4\,\text{ms}^{-1} = 2.875\,\text{ms}^{-1}$ or $2\frac{7}{8}\,\text{ms}^{-1}$.   **A1  A1    3 marks**

**TIP**

Differentiate $V = f(t)$ for acceleration.
Integrate $V = f(t)$ for distance.

**12.** (a)  $\frac{dx}{dt} = 2(1 + t)$, $\frac{dy}{dt} = -2(1 - t)$   **B1  B1**

$\frac{dy}{dx} = \frac{-2(1 - t)}{2(1 + t)} = \frac{t - 1}{t + 1}$   **B1    3 marks**

(b)  At $t = -2$, $\frac{dy}{dx} = 3$ and $x = 1, y = 9$   **M1**

Gradient of normal is $-\frac{1}{3}$   **M1**

Equation of normal $y - 9 = -\frac{1}{3}(x - 1) \Rightarrow x + 3y = 28$   **M1  A1    4 marks**

(c)  $x + 3y = 28$ meets curve again when $(1 + t)^2 + 3(1 - t)^2 = 28$   **M1**

$4t^2 - 4t - 24 = 0 \Rightarrow t^2 - t - 6 = 0$

$(t - 3)(t + 2) = 0$   $\therefore$  line meets curve where $t = 3$   **M1  A1**

That is, at $(16,4)$.   **A1    4 marks**

**TIP**

If you fail to obtain the answers in (a) and (b) still use the results to answer part (c).

**13.** (a)  Volume $= \frac{2}{3}\pi r^3 + \pi r^2 h = 100$   **M1**

$\pi r^2 h = 100 - \frac{2}{3}\pi r^3$   **A1**

$A = 2\pi r^2 + 2\pi rh + \pi r^2$   **M1**

$A = 3\pi r^2 + \frac{2}{r}\left(100 - \frac{2}{3}\pi r^3\right) = \frac{5}{3}\pi r^2 + \frac{200}{r}$   **A1  A1    5 marks**

(b)  $\frac{dA}{dr} = \frac{10\pi r}{3} - \frac{200}{r^2}$   **M1  A1  A1**

$\frac{dA}{dr} = 0$ for minimum $A$, $\frac{10\pi r}{3} - \frac{200}{r^2} = 0$   **M1**

$r = \left(\frac{300}{5\pi}\right)^{\frac{1}{3}} = 2.673\,\text{cm}$   **A1**

Minimum $A = \frac{5}{3}\pi\left(\frac{300}{5\pi}\right)^{\frac{2}{3}} + 200\left(\frac{5\pi}{300}\right)^{\frac{1}{3}}$   **M1**

$= 112.2\,\text{cm}^2$ (to 1 decimal place)   **A1    7 marks**

**TIP**

Remember $V = \frac{2}{3}\pi r^3$ for the hemisphere, $V = \pi r^2 h$ for the cylinder.

**14.** (a) $\begin{cases} u = x^2 & \dfrac{dv}{dx} = \sin x \\[2mm] \dfrac{du}{dx} = 2x & v = -\cos x \end{cases}$ Formula is $\displaystyle \int u\,\dfrac{dv}{dx}\,dx = uv - \int v\,\dfrac{du}{dx}\,dx$ **M1 A1**

$$\int x^2 \sin x\,dx = -x^2 \cos x - \int (-\cos x)2x\,dx \quad \textbf{M1}$$

$$= -x^2 \cos x + 2\int x\cos x\,dx, \text{ as required.} \quad \textbf{A1} \qquad \textbf{4 marks}$$

(b) Now take $\begin{cases} u = x & \dfrac{dv}{dx} = \cos x \\[2mm] \dfrac{du}{dx} = 1 & v = \sin x \end{cases}$ **M1**

$$\int x\cos x\,dx = x\sin x - \int \sin x\,dx = x\sin x + \cos x \quad \textbf{A1 A1}$$

$$\int x^2 \sin x\,dx = -x^2 \cos x + 2x\sin x + 2\cos x + C \quad \textbf{A1} \qquad \textbf{4 marks}$$

(c) Volume of $S = \pi \displaystyle\int x^2 \sin x\,dx$ **M1**

$$= \pi[-x^2 \cos x + 2x\sin x + 2\cos x]_{\frac{\pi}{4}}^{\frac{\pi}{3}} \quad \textbf{A1}$$

$$= \pi\left[-\frac{\pi^2}{9}\times\frac{1}{2} + \frac{2\pi}{3}\times\frac{\sqrt{3}}{2} + 1\right] - \pi\left[-\frac{\pi^2}{16}\times\frac{1}{\sqrt{2}} + \frac{\pi}{2}\times\frac{1}{\sqrt{2}} + \frac{2}{\sqrt{2}}\right]$$

**M1 A1**

$$= 0.555 \text{ (to 3 significant figures)} \quad \textbf{A1} \qquad \textbf{5 marks}$$

**TIP**

Tabulate your work when integrating by parts.

## Solutions to Paper 2 (Pure Mathematics)

**1.** Given $\ln 2 = p, \ln 3 = q$:

(a) $\ln 6 = \ln 2 + \ln 3 = p + q$ **B1** **1 mark**

(b) $\ln\frac{3}{4} = \ln 3 - \ln 4 = \ln 3 - 2\ln 2 = q - 2p$ **B1** **1 mark**

(c) $\ln\left(\dfrac{9e}{8}\right) = \ln 9e - \ln 8 = \ln 3^2 + \ln e - \ln 2^3$ **M1**

$$= 2\ln 3 + 1 - 3\ln 2$$

$$= 2q + 1 - 3p \quad \textbf{A1} \qquad \textbf{2 marks}$$

**TIP**

You need to know the three basic rules of logarithms.

**2.** $(1 - 5x)^8 = 1 + 8(-5x) + \dfrac{8\times7}{1\times2}(-5x)^2 + \dfrac{8\times7\times6}{1\times2\times3}(-5x)^3 + \cdots$ **M1**

$$= 1 - 40x + 700x^2 - 7000x^3 \quad \textbf{A1 A1 A1} \qquad \textbf{4 marks}$$

**TIP**

Do use brackets for the $(-5x)$ terms.

**3.** Using notation in the diagram

$20 = 8\theta$   (arc length $= r\theta$)      **M1**

$\theta = 2.5$   (radians)      **A1**

Using cosine rule in the triangle

$x^2 = 8^2 + 8^2 - 2 \times 8 \times 8 \cos\theta$      **M1**

$= 128 - 128 \cos 2.5$

$= 128 + 102.55 = 230.55$      **M1**

$x = 15.2$ (to 3 significant figures)      $\therefore$   distance $= 15.2\,\text{cm}$      **A1**      **5 marks**

 TIP

Draw a clear sketch.

**4.** (a)      $WX^2 = (4 - 9)^2 + (4 - -1)^2 = 25 + 25 = 50$      **M1**

$XY^2 = (9 - 2)^2 + (-1 - -2)^2 = 49 + 1 = 50$

$\therefore$   $WX = XY$      **A1**      **2 marks**

(b)   Mid-point of $WY = \left(\dfrac{4+2}{2}, \dfrac{4-2}{2}\right) = (3,1)$      **B1**

This is mid-point of $XZ$.

If $Z$ is $(x, y)$, then $\left[\dfrac{x+9}{2}, \dfrac{y-1}{2}\right] \equiv (3, 1)$      **M1**

$x = -3$,      $y = 3$      $\therefore$   $Z$ is $(-3,3)$      **A1**      **3 marks**

 TIP

Note that the mid-points of WY and XZ are the same point.

**5.**          $3(1 - \sin^2 x) = 8 \sin x$

$3 \sin^2 x + 8 \sin x - 3 = 0$      **M1**

$(3 \sin x - 1)(\sin x + 3) = 0 \;\Rightarrow\; \sin x = \dfrac{1}{3}$ or $-3$      **A1**

$\sin x = -3$, has no real solution      **B1**

Answers to 1 decimal place are 19.5°, 160.5°, *none*.      **B1**  **B1**      **5 marks**

 TIP

You need to express cos² x in terms of sin x.

**6.** (a)   $u_n = 2 + \dfrac{2}{u_{n-1} + 1}, u_1 = 1$

$u_2 = 2 + \dfrac{2}{2} = 3$

$u_3 = 2 + \dfrac{2}{3 + 1} = \dfrac{5}{2}$      **B1**

$u_4 = 2 + \dfrac{2}{\frac{5}{2} + 1} = 2 + \dfrac{4}{7} = \dfrac{18}{7}$      **B1**      **2 marks**

(b)   $x = 2 + \dfrac{2}{x + 1} \;\Rightarrow\; x^2 - x - 4 = 0$      **M1**   **A1**

$x = \dfrac{1 + \sqrt{1 + 16}}{2} = \dfrac{1 + \sqrt{17}}{2}.$      **M1**   **A1**      **4 marks**

TIP

Note that answers must be given in correct forms.

7. (a) $y = -1 + 3x - \dfrac{x^2}{4}$

   $\dfrac{dy}{dx} = 3 - \dfrac{x}{2}$  **M1**

   Gradient $= -1$, so $3 - \dfrac{x}{2} = -1 \Rightarrow x = 8$  **M1**  **A1**

   $y = -1 + 3 \times 8 - \dfrac{64}{4} = 7$  **A1**

   $A$ is the point $(8,7)$  **4 marks**

   (b) Gradient of normal at $A$ is 1  **M1**

   Equation of normal is $y - 7 = 1(x - 8)$  **M1**

   that is $x - y - 1 = 0$  **A1**  **3 marks**

TIP

You need to find $\dfrac{dy}{dx}$.

8. $x = 6t^2 - t^3$

   (a) For time of greatest displacement $\dfrac{dx}{dt} = 0$, hence we have $12t - 3t^2 = 0$  **M1**  **A1**

   $t = 4$  **A1**

   When $t = 4$, greatest $x = 6 \times 16 - 64 = 32$

   Greatest displacement $= 32\,\text{m}$  **A1**  **4 marks**

   (b) Greatest speed could occur when $t = 0$ or $t = 6$ or when acceleration is zero.

   Acceleration is 0 when $12 - 6t = 0$, $t = 2$  **M1**

   and speed is then $(24 - 12)\,\text{ms}^{-1} = 12\,\text{ms}^{-1}$  **A1**

   When $t = 6$, speed is $|72 - 108|\,\text{ms}^{-1} = 36\,\text{ms}^{-1}$, which is the greatest speed in the interval.  **M1**  **A1**  **4 marks**

TIP

The greatest (or least) value of the function does not necessarily occur at a stationary point.

9. (a) Ratio of series $= \dfrac{p^2 - p}{p} = p - 1$  **M1**  **A1**

   Third term $= p(p - 1)^2$  **A1**  **3 marks**

   (b) (i) $p = \frac{5}{3}$, so ratio is $\frac{2}{3}$  **B1**

   $S_{15} = \dfrac{\frac{5}{3}[1 - (\frac{2}{3})^{15}]}{1 - \frac{2}{3}}$  **M1**  **A1**

   $= 4.99 \,(\text{to 3 significant figures})$  **A1**  **4 marks**

   (ii) $S_{\infty} = \dfrac{\frac{5}{3}}{1 - \frac{2}{3}} = 5$  **M1**  **A1**  **2 marks**

**10.** (a)   $2(x-3)(x+1) - (x-3)^2 = 4x + 13$

   $2x^2 - 4x - 6 - (x^2 - 6x + 9) = 4x + 13$     **M1**   **B1**

   $x^2 - 2x - 28 = 0$     **A1**

   $(x-1)^2 = 29$ or $x = \dfrac{2 \pm \sqrt{4 + 112}}{2}$     **M1**

   $6.39$ or $-4.39$     **A1**   **A1**     **6 marks**

   (b)   $(x-3)[2x + 2 - x + 3] > 0$     **M1**

   $(x-3)(x+5) > 0$     **M1**   **A1**

   $x > 3$ or $x < -5$     **A1**   **A1**     **5 marks**

**11.** (a)   $\dfrac{\mathrm{d}x}{\mathrm{d}t} = -kx$     **M1**

   $\ln x = -kt + \ln A$, where $\ln A$ is a constant     **A1**

   $x = A\,\mathrm{e}^{-kt}$     **M1**

   $t = 0,\ x = 5000 \ \Rightarrow\ A = 5000$

   $x = 5000\,\mathrm{e}^{-kt}$     **A1**     **4 marks**

   (b)   (i)   $t = 24,\ x = 3000 \ \Rightarrow\ 3000 = 5000\,\mathrm{e}^{-k24}$     **M1**

   $k = \dfrac{1}{24} \ln \dfrac{5}{3} \ (= 0.02128)$     **A1**

   After 36 months, value $= 5000\,\mathrm{e}^{-36k}$     **M1**

   $= £2324$     **A1**     **4 marks**

   (ii)   When value is £1000, $1000 = 5000\,\mathrm{e}^{-kt}$     **M1**

   $\mathrm{e}^{kt} = 5$     **A1**

   $t = \dfrac{\ln 5}{k} = 76$ months     **A1**     **3 marks**

**12.** (a)   $A$ is where $x = 0$ and $B$ is where $y = 0$     **M1**

   At $A$, $y = 2\cos 0 + 1 = 3$     **A1**

   At $B$, $\cos x = -\dfrac{1}{2} \ \Rightarrow\ x = \dfrac{2\pi}{3}$     **A1**     **3 marks**

   (b)   (i)   For area of $R$, $\int (2\cos x + 1)\,\mathrm{d}x$ is required     **M1**

   $\int (2\cos x + 1)\,\mathrm{d}x = 2\sin x + x$     **A1**

   Area of $R = [x + 2\sin x]_0^{\frac{2\pi}{3}} = \dfrac{2\pi}{3} + \sqrt{3}$     **M1**   **A1**     **4 marks**

(ii)   For volume, $\pi \int (2\cos x + 1)^2 \,dx$ is required

$\int (4\cos^2 x + 4\cos x + 1)\,dx$ is required      **M1**

change $4\cos^2 x$ into $2\cos 2x + 2$ using $\cos 2x \equiv 2\cos^2 x - 1$

Volume $= \pi \int (2\cos 2x + 4\cos x + 3)\,dx$      **A1**

$= \pi[\sin 2x + 4\sin x + 3x]_0^{\frac{2\pi}{3}}$      **M1**   **A1**

$= \pi\left(\dfrac{-\sqrt{3}}{2} + 2\sqrt{3} + 2\pi\right) = \pi\left(2\pi + \dfrac{3\sqrt{3}}{2}\right)$      **A1**      **5 marks**

**TIP**

Note that the final answers can include $\pi$ amd $\sqrt{3}$.

13.  $f(x) = \ln x - 8\tan x$

   (a)   $f(6.50) = 0.1096$, $f(6.52) = -0.0559$      **M1**

   f is continuous in $[6.50, 6.52]$ and there is a sign change, so root $\alpha$ lies in the interval.      **A1**      **2 marks**

   (b)   Estimate is where line crosses axis and

   $\alpha \approx 6.50 + p$.      **M1**

   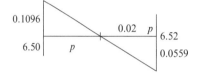

   Similar $\triangle s$ $\dfrac{p}{0.1096} = \dfrac{0.02 - p}{0.0559}$ $\Rightarrow$ $p = 0.0132$

   **M1**   **A1**

   Root $\approx 6.50 + p = 6.5132$ (to 4 decimal places).      **A1**      **4 marks**

   (c)   $f'(x) = \dfrac{1}{x} - 8\sec^2 x$      **M1**   **A1**

   $f(6.50) = 0.1096$, $f'(6.50) = -8.2343$      **A1**

   Newton–Raphson second approximation $= 6.50 + \dfrac{0.1096}{8.2343} = 6.5133$ (to 4 decimal places).

   **M1**   **A1**      **5 marks**

   (d)   Consider $f(6.51315) = 0.00098$, $f(6.51325) = 0.000146$, $f(6.51335) = -0.000683$ and we see sign change in interval $[6.51325, 6.51335]$ $\therefore$ Newton–Raphson approximation is *correct* to 4 decimal places.      **M1**   **A1**      **2 marks**

**TIP**

Draw a sketch to help build up the solution in part (b).

## Solutions to Paper 3 (Pure Mathematics)

1.   $\tan(90° - x) = \dfrac{1}{\sqrt{3}}$ $\Rightarrow$ $\tan(x - 90°) = -\dfrac{1}{\sqrt{3}}$      **M1**

   $\Rightarrow$ $x - 90° = 150°$, $x = 240°$      **M1**   **A1**      **3 marks**

**TIP**

Remember $\tan(-x) = -\tan x$.

**2.** (a) $f(3) = 54 + 9(3 - 2k) - 3(3k + 2) + 6 = 0$    **M1**

        $27k = 81 \implies k = 3$    **A1**    **2 marks**

    (b) $2x^3 - 3x^2 - 11x + 6 = (x - 3)(2x^2 + 3x - 2)$    **M1**   **A1**

        $\implies (x - 3)(2x - 1)(x + 2)$    **A1**    **3 marks**

> **TIP**
>
> Remember that if $(x - a)$ is a factor of $f(x)$ then $f(a) = 0$.

**3.** (a) $T_{1000} = 23 + (1000 - 1)(0.2) = 199.8 + 23 = 222.8$    **M1**   **A1**    **2 marks**

        $S_{240} = \dfrac{240}{2}(46 + 239 \times 0.2) = 11\,256$    **M1**   **A1**   **A1**    **3 marks**

**4.** $\dfrac{x^2 + 12 - 7x}{x} > 0, \quad \dfrac{(x - 4)(x - 3)}{x} > 0$    **M1**   **M1**   **A1**

| $x$ | $-$ | $+$ | $+$ | |
|---|---|---|---|---|
| $x - 3$ | $-$ | $-$ | $+$ | $+$ |
| $x - 4$ | $-$ | $-$ | $-$ | $+$   $+$ |
| $\dfrac{(x - 3)(x - 4)}{x}$ | $-$ | $+$ | $-$ | $+$ |

        0      3      4         **M1**

Solution is $0 < x < 3 \ \bigcup \ x > 4$.    **A1**   **A1**    **6 marks**

> **TIP**
>
> When solving an inequality collect all of the terms on to one side; never cross-multiply.

**5.** (a) (i) $(x + 1)^2 + (y + 2)^2 = 25, \quad (x + 3)^2 + (y - 4)^2 = 1$    **M1**

            Radii are 5 and 1.    **A1**   **A1**    **3 marks**

      (ii) Centres $(-1, -2), (-3, 4) \implies D^2 = (-3 + 1)^2 + (4 + 2)^2$    **M1**

            $D^2 = 40 \quad D = \sqrt{40}$.    **A1**    **2 marks**

    (b) But $r_1 + r_2 = 5 + 1 = 6 < \sqrt{40} \implies$ No intersection.    **A1**    **1 mark**

> **TIP**
>
> (a) Be careful that you obtain the correct signs for the coordinates of the centres of the two circles.
>
> (b) $(x - a)^2 + (y - b)^2 = r^2$ is the equation of a circle centre $(a, b)$, radius $r$.

**6.** (a) $\dfrac{dy}{dx} = 8 - 6x = -4$ when $x = 2$.    **B1**

        Equation of tangent at $(2, 4) \implies y - 4 = -4(x - 2)$    **M1**

        $\implies y = -4x + 12 \equiv y = mx + c, \ m = -4, \ c = 12$    **A1**    **3 marks**

(b)  Gradient of normal $= -\dfrac{1}{-4} = \dfrac{1}{4}$    **B1**

Equation of normal at $(2,4)$  $\Rightarrow$  $y - 4 = \frac{1}{4}(x - 2)$    **M1**

$\Rightarrow A \equiv (-14,0),\ B \equiv (0,3\frac{1}{2})$  $\Rightarrow$  Area $\triangle OAB = 24\frac{1}{2}$    **A1**    **3 marks**

**TIP**

Two lines are perpendicular if the product of their gradients is $-1$.

7.  (a)

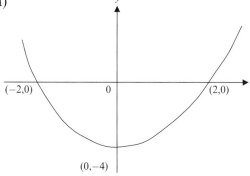

  (b)

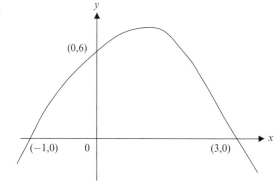

**M1**  Shift
**A1**  coordinates    **2 marks**

**M1**  inverted
**A1**  coordinates    **2 marks**

(c)

**M1**  above $x$-axis
**A1**  coordinates    **2 marks**

**TIP**

Do not forget to indicate the coordinates of the points where the curves cross the coordinate axes.

**8.**

| $x^2$ | 25 | 100 | 225 | 400 | 625 |
|-------|-----|-----|-----|-----|-----|
| $y$ | 149 | 175 | 219 | 280 | 359 |

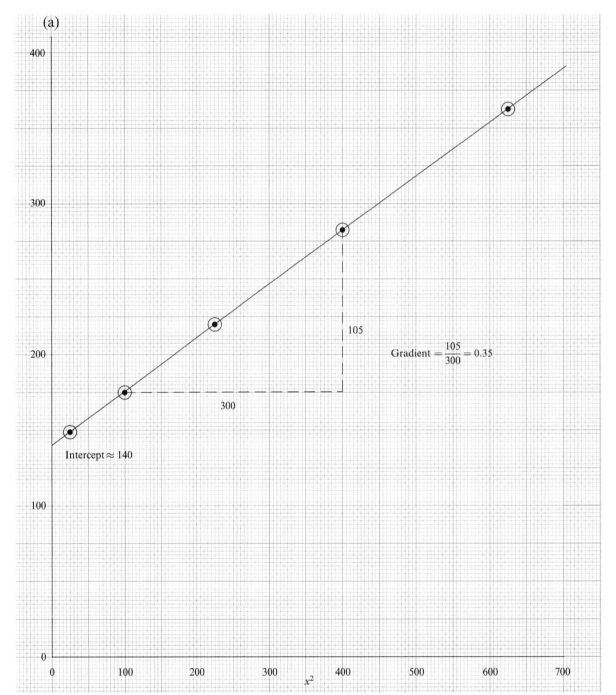

(a)

Intercept $\approx 140$

Gradient $= \dfrac{105}{300} = 0.35$

$x^2$

Straight line graph confirms $y = a + bx^2$    **B1**   **B1**     **2 marks**

(b)   $a =$ intercept on $y$-axis $= 140$     **M1**   **A1**

     $b =$ gradient   $\Rightarrow$   $b = (0.34$ to $0.36)$     **M1**   **A1**      **4 marks**

(c)   $y = 200$,     $x \approx 13$     **B1**     **1 mark**

**TIP**

$y = mx + c$ is the equation of a straight line gradient $m$, intercept on the $y$-axis $(0, c)$.
Do show that you know the meanings of $a$ and $b$.
Do give a table of values of $x^2$; do not just indicate the $x^2$ values by plotting the points.
Always let the examiner know what you are doing. Do not leave the examiner to guess.

**9.** $\dfrac{\mathrm{d}y}{\mathrm{d}t} = \dfrac{(1+x^4)\cdot 2x - x^2\cdot 4x^3}{(1+x^4)^2}$ **M1 A1 A1**

For stationary point $\dfrac{\mathrm{d}y}{\mathrm{d}x} = 0$

$\Rightarrow\ (1+x^4)\cdot 2x - 4x^5 = 0 = 2x - 2x^5$ **M1**

$\Rightarrow\ x(1+x^2)(1-x^2) = x(1+x^2)(1-x)(1+x) = 0$ **A1 A1**

$\Rightarrow\ x = 0, 1$ or $-1$

Stationary points at $(0,0)$, $(1,\tfrac{1}{2})$, $(-1,\tfrac{1}{2})$ **A2** $(1,0)$ **8 marks**

| TIP |
| --- |
| The question asked for the coordinates, so do not leave your answer as $x = 0$, 1 or $-1$. |

**10. (a)** $\displaystyle\int \sin^2\theta\,\mathrm{d}\theta = \int \tfrac{1}{2}(1-\cos 2\theta)\,\mathrm{d}\theta = \tfrac{1}{2}(\theta - \tfrac{1}{2}\sin 2\theta) + C$ **B1 B1** **2 marks**

**(b) (i)** $\displaystyle\int_0^\pi 4\sin x\,\mathrm{d}x = [-4\cos x]_0^\pi = 4 - (-4) = 8$ **M1 A1 A1** **3 marks**

**(ii)** $\pi\displaystyle\int 16\sin^2 x\,\mathrm{d}x = \pi[8(x - \tfrac{1}{2}\sin 2x)]$ **M1 A1**

$\Rightarrow\ \pi\displaystyle\int_0^\pi 16\sin^2 x\,\mathrm{d}x = 8\pi[\pi - 0] = 8\pi^2$ **A1** **3 marks**

| TIP |
| --- |
| A very common mistake in the integration of $\sin x$ and $\cos x$ is to make a sign error. Remember $$\int \sin ax\,\mathrm{d}x = -\frac{1}{a}\cos ax$$ $$\int \cos ax\,\mathrm{d}x = \frac{1}{a}\sin ax.$$ |

**11. (a) (i)** $\sin\theta = \dfrac{r}{R}\ \Rightarrow\ r = R\sin\theta$. **B1** **1 mark**

**(ii)** $R\phi = 2\pi r\ \Rightarrow\ R\phi = 2\pi R\sin\theta\ \Rightarrow\ \phi = 2\pi\sin\theta$. **M1 A1** **2 marks**

**(b)** $V = \tfrac{1}{3}\pi r^2 h = \tfrac{1}{3}\pi r^2 R\cos\theta\ \Rightarrow\ 3V = \pi r^2 R\cos\theta$ **M1**

or $3V = \pi R^3\sin^2\theta\cos\theta$. **A1** **2 marks**

**(c)** $3\dfrac{\mathrm{d}V}{\mathrm{d}\theta} = \pi R^3(2\sin\theta\cos^2\theta - \sin^3\theta)$ **M1 A1 A1**

$= 0$ when $\sin\theta(2\cos^2\theta - \sin^2\theta) = 0$

or $\tan^2\theta = 2$, $\tan\theta = \sqrt{2}$. **M1**

$\tan\theta = \sqrt{2}\ \Rightarrow\ \sin\theta = \sqrt{\left(\dfrac{2}{3}\right)},\ \cos\theta = \dfrac{1}{\sqrt{3}}$ **A1**

$\Rightarrow\ V = \tfrac{1}{3}\pi R^3\cdot\left(\dfrac{2}{3}\right)\left(\dfrac{1}{\sqrt{3}}\right) = \dfrac{2\sqrt{3}}{27}\pi R^3$ **A1** **6 marks**

**(d)** Area $S = \tfrac{1}{2}R^2\phi = \tfrac{1}{2}R^2[2\pi\sqrt{(\tfrac{2}{3})}] = \pi R^2\sqrt{(\tfrac{2}{3})}$ **M1 A1** **2 marks**

| TIP |
| --- |
| The radius $R$ of the circle forms the slant height of the cone. |

**12.** (a)  $\cos 3\theta = \cos 2\theta \cos \theta - \sin 2\theta \sin \theta.$  **B1**

$$= (2\cos^2 \theta - 1)\cos \theta - (2\sin \theta \cos \theta)\sin \theta \qquad \mathbf{M1}$$

$$= (2\cos^2 \theta - 1)\cos \theta - 2(1 - \cos^2 \theta)\cos \theta \qquad \mathbf{M1}$$

$$= 4\cos^3 \theta - 3\cos \theta \qquad \mathbf{A1} \qquad \textbf{4 marks}$$

(b)  $2\cos 3\theta = \left(x + \dfrac{1}{x}\right)^3 - 3\left(x + \dfrac{1}{x}\right) \qquad \mathbf{M1}$

$$= \left(x^3 + 3x + \dfrac{3}{x} + \dfrac{1}{x^3}\right) - 3\left(x + \dfrac{1}{x}\right) \qquad \mathbf{A1}$$

$$= x^3 + \dfrac{1}{x^3} \qquad \mathbf{A1} \qquad \textbf{3 marks}$$

(c)  $\cos 3\theta = 1 - \dfrac{9\theta^2}{2!} + \dfrac{81\theta^4}{4!}, \qquad \cos \theta = 1 - \dfrac{\theta^2}{2!} + \dfrac{\theta^4}{4!} \qquad \mathbf{B1}$

$$\Rightarrow \quad \cos^3 \theta = \dfrac{1}{4}(\cos 3\theta + 3\cos \theta)$$

$$= \dfrac{1}{4}\left[\left(1 - \dfrac{9\theta^2}{2!} + \dfrac{81\theta^4}{4!}\right) + 3\left(1 - \dfrac{\theta^2}{2!} + \dfrac{\theta^4}{4!}\right)\right] \qquad \mathbf{M1}$$

$$= 1 - \dfrac{3\theta^2}{2} + \dfrac{7}{8}\theta^4. \qquad \mathbf{A1} \qquad \textbf{3 marks}$$

(d)  When  $\theta = \dfrac{\pi}{10} \qquad \cos^3 \theta = 1 - \dfrac{3\pi^2}{200} + \dfrac{7}{8} \cdot \dfrac{\pi^4}{10,000}$

$$\approx 0.86047923 \qquad \mathbf{B1}$$

But  $\cos^3\left(\dfrac{\pi}{10}\right) \approx 0.8602387 \qquad \mathbf{B1}$

$$\Rightarrow \quad \text{Relative error} = \dfrac{0.00024053}{0.8602387}$$

$$\approx 0.0002796 \qquad \mathbf{B1} \qquad \textbf{3 marks}$$

> **TIP**
>
> Remember  $\cos(A + B) = \cos A \cos B - \sin A \sin B.$

**13.** (a)  $3x^2 + 6y^2 \dfrac{dy}{dx} + \left(3y + 3x \dfrac{dy}{dx}\right) = 0 \qquad \mathbf{B1} \quad \mathbf{M1} \quad \mathbf{A1} \quad \mathbf{M1} \quad \mathbf{A1}$

$$\Rightarrow \quad \dfrac{dy}{dx} = -\dfrac{3(x^2 + y)}{3(2y^2 + x)} = -\dfrac{3}{4} \qquad \mathbf{A1} \qquad \textbf{6 marks}$$

(b)  $\dfrac{dx}{dt} = 2e^{2t}\cos 2t - 2e^{2t}\sin 2t \qquad \mathbf{M1} \quad \mathbf{A1} \text{ (der. } e^{2t}\text{)} \quad \mathbf{A1} \text{ (der. } \sin 2t\text{)} \quad \mathbf{A1} \text{ (der. } \cos 2t\text{)}$

$$\dfrac{dy}{dt} = 2e^{2t}\sin 2t + 2e^{2t}\cos 2t$$

$$\Rightarrow \quad \dfrac{dy}{dx} = \dfrac{\sin 2t + \cos 2t}{\cos 2t - \sin 2t} = \dfrac{1 + \tan 2t}{1 - \tan 2t} \qquad \mathbf{M1} \quad \mathbf{A1} \quad \mathbf{A1}$$

$$= \dfrac{\tan \dfrac{\pi}{4} + \tan 2t}{1 - \tan \dfrac{\pi}{4} \tan 2t} = \tan\left(\dfrac{\pi}{4} + 2t\right) \qquad \mathbf{A1} \qquad \textbf{8 marks}$$

> **TIP**
>
> (a)  Use  $\dfrac{d}{dx}(y^n) = \dfrac{dy}{dx} \cdot \dfrac{d}{dy}(y^n).$
>
> (b)  Use  $\dfrac{dy}{dx} = \left(\dfrac{dy}{dt}\right) \bigg/ \left(\dfrac{dx}{dt}\right)$ ; also remember that  $\tan \dfrac{\pi}{4} = 1.$

## Solutions to Paper 4 (Pure Mathematics)

1. Greatest possible length $= \dfrac{75945}{100.5} \Rightarrow 756\,\text{m}$ **B1 B1 M1 A1**  **4 marks**

> **TIP**
>
> You need the maximum area and the minimum width.

2. $2x - 30° = 180° - (x - 40°) \Rightarrow x = 83\frac{1}{3}°$ **M1 A1**

   $2x - 30° = 360° + (x - 40°) \Rightarrow x = 350°$ **M1 A1**  **4 marks**

> **TIP**
>
> $\sin x = \sin y$ implies $x = y$ or $x = 180° - y$ or $x = 360° + y$, etc.

3. $\dfrac{a}{1-r} = 8,\ \dfrac{a}{1-r^2} = 6$  **M1 A1**

   Dividing $\dfrac{1-r^2}{1-r} = \dfrac{8}{6} \Rightarrow 1 + r = \dfrac{4}{3} \qquad r = \dfrac{1}{3}$  **M1 A1**

   Substituting $a = 8 \times \dfrac{2}{3} = 5\dfrac{1}{3}$  **A1**  **5 marks**

> **TIP**
>
> Remember the formula for the sum to infinity of the infinite geometric series.

4. $(x - a)(x - a - 1) \equiv x^2 + px + q \equiv x^2 - x(2a + 1) + a(a + 1)$  **M1 A1**

   Comparing coefficients $p = -(2a + 1), q = a(a + 1)$  **M1**

   Eliminating $a \Rightarrow p^2 = 4a^2 + 4a + 1 = 4a(a + 1) + 1$  **M1 A1**

   $\Rightarrow p^2 = 4q + 1$  **5 marks**

> **TIP**
>
> Many candidates answering this question would immediately think of using the formula $\dfrac{-b \pm \sqrt{(b^2 - 4ac)}}{2a}$ for the roots of the equation $x^2 + px + q = 0$. This could involve more complicated algebraic manipulation. It is usually advisable to avoid square root signs if possible.
>
> Roots $\Rightarrow a = \dfrac{-p - \sqrt{(p^2 - 4q)}}{2},\quad a + 1 = \dfrac{-p + \sqrt{(p^2 - 4q)}}{2}$
>
> Subtracting $1 = \sqrt{(p^2 - 4q)}$
>
> Squaring $1 = p^2 - 4q \Rightarrow p^2 = 4q + 1$

5. (a) $\angle ACB = 180° - (45.6° + 63.1°) = 71.3°$  **M1 A1**

   $AC = \dfrac{89 \sin 63.1°}{\sin 71.3°} = 83.8\,\text{m}$  **M1 A1**  **4 marks**

   (b) Width of canal $= AC \sin 45.6° = 59.9\,\text{m}$  **M1 A1**  **2 marks**

> **TIP**
>
> Remember the sum of the angles of a triangle is 180°.

**6.** $x^2 + 2x - 3 = 2 \Rightarrow (x+1)^2 = 6 \qquad x = -1 \pm \sqrt{6}$ **M1 A1**

$x^2 + 2x - 3 = -2 \Rightarrow (x+1)^2 = 2 \qquad x = -1 \pm \sqrt{2}$ **M1 A1**

$-1 + \sqrt{2} < x < -1 + \sqrt{6} \;\cup\; -1 - \sqrt{6} < x < -1 - \sqrt{2}$ **M1 A1 A1** **7 marks**

**TIP**

$|f(x)| = 2$ implies $f(x) = \pm 2$.

**7.** (a) $(x + 2y)^6 = x^6 + 6x^5(2y) + 15x^4(2y)^2 + 20x^3(2y)^3 + 15x^2(2y)^4$

$\qquad = (x^6 + 12x^5 y) + (60x^4 y^2 + 160x^3 y^3) + 240x^2 y^4$ **B1 B1 B1** **3 marks**

(b) $x = 1,\ y = 0.01$ **M1 A1**

$\Rightarrow (1.02)^6 = 1 + 0.12 + 0.006 + 0.00016 + 0.0000024$ **A1**

$= 1.1262.$ **A1** **4 marks**

**TIP**

Place brackets around $(2y)$ to avoid expansion errors.

**8.** (a) $r = h \tan\theta \Rightarrow A = \pi r^2 = \pi h^2 \tan^2\theta.$ **B1** **1 mark**

(b) $V = \tfrac{1}{3}\pi r^2 h \Rightarrow V = \tfrac{1}{3}\pi h^2 \tan^2\theta \cdot h = \tfrac{1}{3}\pi h^3 \tan^2\theta.$ **B1** **1 mark**

(c) $\dfrac{dV}{dt} = k \qquad \dfrac{dV}{dh} = \dfrac{1}{3}\pi \cdot 3h^2 \tan^2\theta = \pi h^2 \tan^2\theta$ **M1 A1**

$\dfrac{dh}{dt} = \dfrac{dh}{dV}\dfrac{dV}{dt} = \dfrac{1}{\pi h^2 \tan^2\theta} \cdot k = \dfrac{k}{\pi r^2}$ **M1 A1** **4 marks**

(d) $A = \pi h^2 \tan^2\theta \Rightarrow \dfrac{dA}{dh} = 2\pi h \tan^2\theta$ **B1**

$\dfrac{dA}{dt} = \dfrac{dA}{dh} \cdot \dfrac{dh}{dt} = 2\pi h \tan^2\theta \cdot \dfrac{k}{\pi r^2}$ **M1**

$= 2h \tan^2\theta \left( \dfrac{k}{h^2 \tan^2\theta} \right) = \dfrac{2k}{h}$ **A1** **3 marks**

**TIP**

If you cannot prove the formulae for $A$ and $V$ use the values given in the question in order to complete the remainder of the question.

**9.** (a) $\dfrac{dx}{dt} = 4 - \dfrac{2}{2t}; \qquad \dfrac{dy}{dt} = 2t - \dfrac{2t}{t^2}$ **M1 A1 A1**

$\dfrac{dy}{dx} = \dfrac{dy}{dt} \cdot \dfrac{dt}{dx} = \dfrac{2t^3 - 2t}{t^2} \cdot \dfrac{2t}{8t - 2} = \dfrac{2(t^2 - 1)}{4t - 1}$ **M1 A1** **5 marks**

(b) $\dfrac{dy}{dx} = \dfrac{1}{2}$ when $4(t^2 - 1) = 4t - 1$ **M1**

$\Rightarrow 4t^2 - 4t - 3 = 0 = (2t + 1)(2t - 3),\ t = -\tfrac{1}{2}$ or $\tfrac{3}{2}$ **A1**

But $t > 0 \Rightarrow t = \tfrac{3}{2}$ **A1** **3 marks**

(c) $A = (6 - \ln 3,\ \tfrac{9}{4} - \ln(\tfrac{9}{4}))$ **A1**

Equation of tangent $y - \tfrac{9}{4} + \ln(\tfrac{9}{4}) = \tfrac{1}{2}(x - 6 + \ln 3)$ **M1 A1**

$\Rightarrow 4y = 2x - 3 + \ln\left( \dfrac{4^4}{9^3} \right)$ **A1** **4 marks**

**TIP**

Remember, the equation of a straight line through the point $(x_1, y_1)$ gradient $m$ is given by $y - y_1 = m(x - x_1)$.

The final part asks for an equation of the tangent in its simplest form. Any form equivalent to the above answer would be acceptable as long as the constants and the logarithmic terms are collected. For example:

$$y = \tfrac{1}{2}x - \tfrac{3}{4} + \tfrac{1}{4}\ln\left(\frac{256}{729}\right).$$

**10.** (a)   $A(x^2 + 4) + (Bx + C)(x + 1) \equiv x^2 + 2x - 4$

$x = -1 \Rightarrow A = -1$   **B1**

$x^2$ coefficients $\Rightarrow A + B = 1 \Rightarrow B = 2$   **B1**

constants $\Rightarrow 4A + C = -4 \Rightarrow C = 0$   **B1**

$$\int_1^4 \left(\frac{-1}{x+1} + \frac{2x}{x^2+4}\right) dx = [-\ln(x+1) + \ln(x^2+4)]_1^4 \quad \textbf{B1} \quad \textbf{B1}$$

$$= \ln 20 - \ln 5 + \ln 2 - \ln 5 = \ln\left(\frac{40}{25}\right) = \ln\left(\frac{8}{5}\right) \quad \textbf{M1} \quad \textbf{A1} \qquad \textbf{7 marks}$$

(b)   $\displaystyle\int 1 \ln x \, dx = x \ln x - \int x \cdot \frac{1}{x} \, dx = x \ln x - x + C$   **M1** **A1** **A1**

Separating the variables $\Rightarrow \displaystyle\int \cos 2y \, dy = \int \ln x \, dx$   **M1**

$\Rightarrow \tfrac{1}{2} \sin 2y = x \ln x - x + C$ is the general solution.   **A1** **A1**   **6 marks**

**TIP**

Do not forget that the answer to part (a) had to be left in the form $\ln\left(\dfrac{A}{B}\right)$.

In (b), take $u = \ln x$ and $\dfrac{dv}{dx} = 1$ when integrating by parts.

**11.** (a)   Sketch   **B1**

coordinates $(0, -9)$, $(3, 0)$   **B1**   **2 marks**

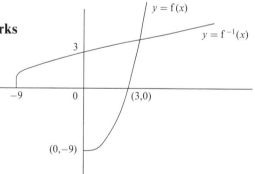

(c)   Sketch   **B1**

coordinates   **B1**   **2 marks**

(b)   $y = x^2 - 9 \Rightarrow x = y^2 - 9 \Rightarrow y = \pm\sqrt{x+9}$   **M1**   **A1**

$f^{-1}: x \mapsto \sqrt{x+9} \quad x \in \mathbb{R}, x \geqslant -9$   **A1**

Domain $x \geqslant 9$, Range $y \geqslant 0$   **B1** **B1**   **5 marks**

(d)   $x^2 - 9 = 4x \Rightarrow (x-2)^2 = 13 \quad x = 2 + \sqrt{13}$   **M1**   **A1**   **2 marks**

(e)   Curves $y = f(x)$ and $y = f^{-1}(x)$ intersect on $y = x$   **M1**

$\Rightarrow x^2 - 9 = x$  or  $(x - \tfrac{1}{2})^2 = 9\tfrac{1}{4}$   **M1**

$\Rightarrow x = \tfrac{1}{2} \pm \sqrt{9\tfrac{1}{4}}$  Required root is $\tfrac{1}{2} + \sqrt{9\tfrac{1}{4}}$

i.e. $x = 3.54$ (to 3 significant figures)   **A1**   **3 marks**

**TIP**

Follow all of the instructions regarding the required form of the answers.
Do make sure you draw both graph sketches using the same axes.
Do make sure you state the coordinates $(0,-9)$, $(3,0)$ – the wording of the question means it is not sufficient simply to show the 3 and $-9$ on the axes.

**12.** (a) $\dfrac{6}{x} = 9 - 3x \Rightarrow 3x^2 - 9x + 6 = 0 = 3(x-1)(x-2)$    **M1**   **M1**

$A \equiv (1,6)$, $B \equiv (2,3)$    **A1**   **A1**    **4 marks**

(b) Area $\Rightarrow \displaystyle\int \left(9 - 3x - \dfrac{6}{x}\right) dx = \left(9x - \dfrac{3x^2}{2}\right) - 6\ln x$    **M1**   **A1**   **A1**

$\displaystyle\int_1^2 = (18 - 6 - 6\ln 2) - (9 - \tfrac{3}{2}) = 4\tfrac{1}{2} - 6\ln 2$    **M1\***   **A1**    **5 marks**

(c) Volume $\Rightarrow \pi \displaystyle\int (9 - 3x)^2 \, dx - \pi \int \dfrac{36}{x^2} \, dx$    **M1** (either)   **M1**

$= \pi \dfrac{(9 - 3x)^3}{3(-3)} + \dfrac{\pi \cdot 36}{x}$    **A1**   **A1**

$\displaystyle\int_1^2 = \pi \left[\dfrac{3^3}{-9} + \dfrac{36}{2} + \dfrac{6^3}{+9} - 36\right]$

(\* if **M1** for correct use of limits is not earned earlier it can be earned here.)

$= 3\pi$    **A1**    **5 marks**

**TIP**

In part (c) do NOT use $\pi \int (y_1 - y_2)^2 \, dx$, it's completely wrong.

## Solutions to Paper 5 (Statistics)

**1.** (a) (i) A census is used to gather data about a whole population.    **B1**    **1 mark**

(ii) A sample survey is used to gather data from some members of a population who are intended to be representative of the whole population.    **B1**    **1 mark**

(b) *Example of a census*: Every student in the Sixth Form college is asked how much he or she earns each week through part-time work.    **B1**

*Example of a sample survey*: Every 10th student on the entire college list is asked how much he or she earns each week in part-time work.    **B1**    **2 marks.**

**TIP**

Many correct examples are possible.

**2.** (a) Mean $= \dfrac{354}{20} = 17.7$    **M1**   **A1**    **2 marks**

(b) Variance $= 6.91$ (from calculator)    **M1**   **A1**

S.D. $= 2.63$    **A1**    **3 marks**

**TIP**

Double-check your answers from a calculator.
Make sure that you fully understand how to use the statistical functions on your calculator to find means and variances and hence standard deviations.

3. Draw a tree diagram, as shown, to illustrate the data and the probabilities.

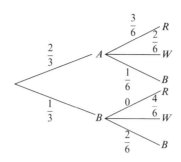

(a) $P$ (white ball is drawn) $= \dfrac{2}{3} \times \dfrac{2}{6} + \dfrac{1}{3} \times \dfrac{4}{6} = \dfrac{8}{18} = \dfrac{4}{9}$    **M1   A1   A1      3 marks**

(b) $P(A \text{ used} \mid \text{white ball obtained}) = \dfrac{P(A \cap W)}{P(W)} = \dfrac{\frac{2}{3} \times \frac{2}{6}}{\frac{8}{18}} = \dfrac{1}{2}$

**M1   A1   M1   A1   4 marks**

> **TIP**
>
> Use a tree diagram to show the sample space.

4. Standard Error of the mean $= \dfrac{19.3}{\sqrt{120}} = 1.762$    **M1   A1   A1**

   95% confidence interval is $47.5 \pm 1.762 \times \mathbf{1.96}$    **M1   B1**

   Lower limit $= 44.05 \approx 44$    **A1**

   Upper limit $= 50.95 \approx 51$    **A1**

   Interval is $(44, 51)$    **7 marks**

> **TIP**
>
> 120 is considered to be a large sample.

5. (a) $P(5 \text{ calls to } A) = e^{-4} \times \dfrac{4^5}{5!} \approx 0.16$ (to 2 significant figures)    **M1   A1      2 marks**

   (b) $P(\text{at least 3 calls to } B) = 1 - P(0) - P(1) - P(2)$    **M1**

   $= 1 - e^{-5} - 5e^{-5} - \dfrac{5^2}{2}e^{-5}$    **A1**

   $= 0.88$ (to 2 significant figures)    **A1      3 marks**

   (c) $P(3 \text{ calls to } A \text{ and } B \text{ together})$

   | | $A$ | $B$ | Probability |
   |---|---|---|---|
   | Calls | 0 | 3 | $e^{-4} \times e^{-5} \times \dfrac{5^3}{3!}$ |
   | | 1 | 2 | $4e^{-4} \times e^{-5} \times \dfrac{5^2}{2}$ |
   | | 2 | 1 | $\dfrac{4^2}{2}e^{-4} \times e^{-5} \times 5$ |
   | | 3 | 0 | $\dfrac{4^3}{3!} \times e^{-4} \times e^{-5}$    **M1   A1** |

Sum of probabilities $= P$ (3 calls to $A$ and $B$ in all)

$= 0.015$ (to 2 significant figures)  **A1**    **3 marks**

**TIP**

You can use cumulative Poisson tables if you wish.

**6.** (a) For samples of 1000 women, the proportion intending to buy the product will have a

$N\left(x, \dfrac{x(1-x)}{1000}\right)$ distribution    **M1**

where $x$ is the true, but unknown, population proportion. We take the sample proportion 0.357 as an estimate for $x$. A 95% confidence interval contains those hypothetical values of $x$ which we would not be able to reject on the basis of this sample. That is:

$-1.96 < \dfrac{0.357 - x'}{\sqrt{\dfrac{0.357 \times (1-0.357)}{1000}}} < 1.96$    **M1  A1**

where $x'$ is the hypothetical value of $x$.

$0.357 - 1.96\sqrt{\dfrac{0.357 \times 0.643}{1000}} < x' < 0.357 + 1.96\sqrt{\dfrac{0.357 \times 0.643}{1000}}$    **M1**

$0.33 < x' < 0.39$ is the required interval.    **A1  A1**    **6 marks**

(b) If 20 such surveys were done, we would expect 95% of them, that is, 19, to produce a confidence interval enclosing the true value of $x$.    **M1  A1**    **2 marks**

**7.** (a)

| $J_1$ | 1 | 2 | 3 | 4 | 5 | 6 | 7 | 8 | 9 | 10 |
|-------|---|---|---|---|---|---|---|---|---|----|
| $J_2$ | 2 | 6 | 4 | 3 | 1 | 7 | 5 | 10 | 8 | 9 |
| $|d|$ | 1 | 4 | 1 | 1 | 4 | 1 | 2 | 2 | 1 | 1 |
| $d^2$ | 1 | 16 | 1 | 1 | 16 | 1 | 4 | 4 | 1 | 1 |

$\sum d^2 = 46$    **M1  A1**

Spearman's coefficient, $r_s = 1 - \dfrac{6\sum d^2}{n(n^2-1)} = 1 - \dfrac{6 \times 46}{10(10^2-1)} = 0.7212$

**M1  A1  A1**    **5 marks**

(b) $\left.\begin{array}{l} H_0: \rho = 0 \\ H_1: \rho \neq 0 \end{array}\right\}$ $r_s > 0.5636 \Rightarrow$ At 5% level, result is significant.    **B1  M1  A1**

$\left.\begin{array}{l} H_0: \rho = 0 \\ H_1: \rho \neq 0 \end{array}\right\}$ $r_s < 0.7455 \Rightarrow$ At 1% level, result is *NOT* significant.

**B1  A1**    **5 marks**

**TIP**

Tabulate your work clearly and do show all of your working.

**8.** (a) $k(1 + 3 + 5 + 7 + 9) = 1 \Rightarrow k = \frac{1}{25}$    **M1  A1**    **2 marks**

(b)

| $X$ | 1 | 3 | 5 | 7 | 9 |
|-----|---|---|---|---|---|
| $P(X = x)$ | $\frac{1}{25}$ | $\frac{3}{35}$ | $\frac{5}{25}$ | $\frac{7}{25}$ | $\frac{9}{25}$ |

$E(X) = 1 \times \frac{1}{25} + 3 \times \frac{3}{25} + 5 \times \frac{5}{25} + 7 \times \frac{7}{25} + 9 \times \frac{9}{25}$    **M1  A1**

$= 6.6$    **A1**    **3 marks**

(c) $\text{Var}(X) = 1^2 \times \frac{1}{25} + 3^2 \times \frac{3}{25} + 5^2 \times \frac{5}{25} + 7^2 \times \frac{7}{25} + 9^2 \times \frac{9}{25} - (6.6)^2$    **M1**    **A1**

$= 5.44$    **A1**    **3 marks**

(d) $\text{Var}(2X - 4) = 2^2 \cdot \text{Var}(X)$    **M1**    **A1**

$= 21.76$    **A1**    **3 marks**

> **TIP**
>
> Learn the formulae required and remember $\sum P(x) = 1$.

9. (a) 1   Only two possible outcomes, 'success' and 'failure'.

     2   Each trial is independent of the other trials.

     3   Each trial involves a constant probability $P$ of success.

     4   There is a fixed number of trials.    **B1**    1 correct,    **B1**    further 1 correct    **2 marks**

(b) (i) $P(\text{all germinate}) = 0.9^{12} = 0.282 \,(\text{to 3 significant figures})$    **M1**    **A1**    **2 marks**

     (ii) $P(10 \text{ germinate}) = \binom{12}{10} 0.9^{10}(0.1)^2$    **M1**

$= 66 \times 0.9^{10} \times 0.01$    **A1**

$= 0.230 \,(\text{to 3 significant figures})$    **A1**    **3 marks**

     (iii) $P(\text{at least 10 germinate})$

$= \text{ANS. (a)} + \text{ANS. (b)} + \binom{12}{11} 0.9^{11}(0.1)$    **M1**    **A1**

$= 0.889 \,(\text{to 3 significant figures})$    **M1**    **A1**    **4 marks**

> **TIP**
>
> Be careful not to lose accuracy through premature approximation.

10. Let weight of powder be $X$ (in grams)

Let weight of packet be $Y$ (in grams)

Then $X$ is $N(625,225)$ and $Y$ is $N(25,9)$

(a) $X + Y$ is $N(650,234)$    **M1**    **A1**

$P(X + Y > 630) = P\left(Z > \dfrac{630 - 650}{\sqrt{234}}\right)$    **M1**

$= P(Z > -1.307)$    **A1**

$= 1 - P(Z > 1.307) = 0.9045$    **M1**    **A1**    **6 marks**

(b) $X_1 + X_2 + X_3 + X_4 = N(2500,900)$    **M1**    **A1**

$P(X_1 + X_2 + X_3 + X_4 > 2450) = P\left(Z > \dfrac{2450 - 2500}{\sqrt{900}}\right)$    **M1**

$= P(Z > -1\tfrac{2}{3})$    **A1**

$= 1 - P(Z > 1\tfrac{2}{3}) = 0.9522$    **M1**    **A1**    **6 marks**

> **TIP**
>
> Use a sketch to help you evaluate normal integral approximations from the tables.

**11.** (a)   Sketch    **B2**    **2 marks**

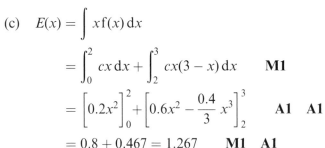

(b)   Total area = 1

$\Rightarrow\ 2c + \frac{1}{2} \times 1 \times c = 1$

$c = 0.4$    **M1**   **A1**    **2 marks**

(c)   $E(x) = \int x f(x)\,dx$

$$= \int_0^2 cx\,dx + \int_2^3 cx(3-x)\,dx \qquad \textbf{M1}$$

$$= \left[0.2x^2\right]_0^2 + \left[0.6x^2 - \frac{0.4}{3}x^3\right]_2^3 \qquad \textbf{A1}\quad\textbf{A1}$$

$$= 0.8 + 0.467 = 1.267 \qquad \textbf{M1}\quad\textbf{A1}$$

Median, $m$, is such that $\displaystyle\int_{-\infty}^{m} f(x)\,dx = 0.5$ and clearly    **M1**

$m < 2$ from sketch so $mc = 0.5$ and $c = 0.4$

$\Rightarrow\ m = \dfrac{5}{4} = 1.25$    **M1**   **A1**    **8 marks**

(d)   $\mathrm{Var}(X) = \displaystyle\int_{-\infty}^{\infty} x^2 f(x)\,dx - [E(X)]^2$    **M1**

$$= \int_0^2 0.4x^2\,dx + \int_2^3 (1.2x^2 - 0.4x^3)\,dx - 1.267^2 \qquad \textbf{A1}$$

$$= \left[\frac{0.4}{3}x^3\right]_0^2 + \left[0.4x^3 - 0.1x^4\right]_2^3 - 1.267^2 \qquad \textbf{A1}$$

$$= 1.067 + 10.8 - 8.1 - 3.2 + 1.6 - 1.604 = 0.561 \qquad \textbf{M1}\quad\textbf{A1}\qquad\textbf{5 marks}$$

**TIP**

Do learn the required formulae and do show all of your working.

## Solutions to Paper 6 (Statistics)

**1.** (a)   1   There is a fixed number of trials.

2   The trials are independent.

3   There is a constant probability $p$ of success at each trial.

4   Only two outcomes, 'success' and 'failure' are possible at each trial.

5   The variable is the total number of successes in $n$ trials.

**B1** for any two; **B1** for further two; **B1** for final one     Maximum **3 marks**

(b)   (i)   Yes, the binomial distribution is suitable.    **B1**

$n = 10, \qquad p = \frac{1}{6}$    **B1**

(ii)   No, the binomial distribution is not a suitable model.    **B1**

(iii)   Yes, the binomial distribution is suitable.    **B1**

$n = 500, \qquad p = \frac{1}{7}.$    **B1**    **5 marks**

**TIP**

Make sure you state all of the conditions.

**2.** (a) (i) $\mu = \dfrac{315}{30} = 10.5$    **M1**   **A1**    **2 marks**

    (ii) $\sigma = \sqrt{\dfrac{3350}{30} - 10.5^2} = 1.19$    **M1**   **A1**    **2 marks**

  (b) (i) Mean would be unaffected (**B1**) due to symmetry of 9 and 12 about the previous calculated mean.    **B1**    **2 marks**

    (ii) The standard deviation would increase (**B1**). Both 9 and 12 have deviations from the mean greater than 1.19, resulting in a greater spread.    **B1**    **2 marks**

> **TIP**
>
> Do not use a calculator just stating single answers. Show your working in order to cover the method marks.

**3.** $\hat{p}_\omega = \dfrac{41}{66}$    $\hat{p}_m = \dfrac{14}{34}$   $\Rightarrow$   $\hat{p}_\omega - \hat{p}_m = \dfrac{41}{66} - \dfrac{14}{34}$    **B1**   **M1**   **A1**

$\Rightarrow \dfrac{41}{66} - \dfrac{14}{34} \pm 1.96 \sqrt{\dfrac{\frac{41}{66} \times \frac{25}{66}}{66} + \dfrac{\frac{14}{34} \times \frac{20}{34}}{34}}$    **M1**   **A1**   **A1**

$\Rightarrow 0.62121 - 0.41176 \pm 1.96\sqrt{0.00357 + 0.00712}$

$\Rightarrow 0.20945 \pm 0.020265$

$(0.2297, 0.1892)$    **A1**   **A1**    **8 marks**

> **TIP**
>
> Remember you are concerned with the *difference* between the proportions of men and women.

**4.** (a) $\Phi(Z) = 0.9$    $Z = 1.282$    **B1**

    $\Rightarrow \dfrac{153.2 - \mu}{\sigma} = 1.282$    **M1**   **A1**

    $\Phi(Z) = 0.2$    $Z = -0.842$    **B1**

    $\Rightarrow \dfrac{138.6 - \mu}{\sigma} = -0.842.$    **A1**    **5 marks**

  (b) Solving $(153 - \mu)(0.842) = (\mu - 138.6)1.282$    **M1**

    $\Rightarrow 2.123\mu = 306.541 \Rightarrow \mu = 144.39$    **A1**

    $\sigma = 6.87$    **A1**    **3 marks**

> **TIP**
>
> Make sure you know how to read $Z$ from the table giving $\Phi(Z)$.

**5.** $E(X - Y) = 19 - 18.6 = 0.4$    **M1**   **A1**

$\operatorname{Var}(X - Y) = 0.02 + 0.01 = 0.03$    **M1**   **A1**

$X - Y \sim N(0.4, 0.03)$

$Z = \dfrac{0 - 0.4}{\sqrt{0.03}} = -2.3094$    **M1**   **A1**

$$P(Z < 0) = \Phi(-2.3094) = 1 - \Phi(2.3094) \quad \textbf{M1} \quad \textbf{A1}$$

$$= 1 - 0.98954 = 0.01046$$

$\Rightarrow$ 1.04% will not fit.    **A1**    **9 marks**

**TIP**

Remember $E(X - Y) = E(X) - E(Y)$, $\text{Var}(X - Y) = \text{Var}(X) + \text{Var}(Y)$.

**6.**

| | | Value | Probability | Expectation | | | |
|---|---|---|---|---|---|---|---|
| | | **Value** | **Probability** | **Expectation** | **M1** | **M1** | **M1** |
| R | R | $6 + 6$ | $\frac{1}{2} \times \frac{1}{2}$ | $\frac{1}{4} \times 12 = 3$ | **A1** | | |
| R | B | $6 - 72$ | $\frac{1}{2} \times \frac{1}{3}$ | $\frac{1}{6}(-66) = -11$ | **A1** | | |
| B | R | | | $= -11$ | | | |
| B | B | $-72 - 72$ | $\frac{1}{3} \times \frac{1}{3}$ | $\frac{1}{9}(-144) = -16$ | **A1** | | |
| R | G | $6 + 180$ | $\frac{1}{2} \times \frac{1}{6}$ | $\frac{1}{12} \times 186 = 15\frac{1}{2}$ | **A1** | | |
| G | R | | | $= 15\frac{1}{2}$ | | | |
| B | G | $-72 + 180$ | $\frac{1}{3} \times \frac{1}{6}$ | $\frac{1}{18} \times 108 = 6$ | **A1** | | |
| G | B | | | $= 6$ | | | |
| G | G | $180 + 180$ | $\frac{1}{6} \times \frac{1}{6}$ | $\frac{1}{36} \times 360 = 10$ | **A1** | | |

Total $= -38 + 56 = 18$

Cost of game $= 20$

Total Expectation $= 18 - 20 = -2$.    **A1**    **10 marks**

**TIP**

Make sure you take every possible throw into account.

**7.** (a)

| | A | B | C | D | E | F | G | H | I | J | K | L | M | N | O | |
|---|---|---|---|---|---|---|---|---|---|---|---|---|---|---|---|---|
| d | 2 | 4 | 3 | 3 | 3 | 3 | 0 | 1 | 2 | 5 | 2 | 3 | 3 | 6 | 2 | **B1** |
| $d^2$ | 4 | 16 | 9 | 9 | 9 | 9 | 0 | 1 | 4 | 25 | 4 | 9 | 9 | 36 | 4 | **B1** |

$$r_s = 1 - \frac{6 \sum d^2}{n(n^2 - 1)} = 1 - \frac{6 \times 148}{15(15^2 - 1)} \quad \textbf{M1} \quad \textbf{A1}$$

$$= 1 - 0.2643 \approx 0.736 \quad \textbf{A1} \quad \textbf{5 marks}$$

(b)   $H_0$: $\rho = 0$   No correlation.    **B1**

    $H_1$: $\rho > 0$   Results positively correlated.    **B1**

    Total size 15   $\Rightarrow$   5% $= 0.5214 < 0.736$    **B1**   **M1**

    $\Rightarrow$ result is significant

    $\Rightarrow$ Reject $H_0$ accept $H_1$

    Results positively correlated.    **A1**    **5 marks**

**TIP**

Tabulate your working and state clearly your hypotheses.

8. (a) $\displaystyle\int_0^4 \left( K - \frac{1}{16}x^2 \right) dx = \left[ Kx - \frac{1}{48}x^3 \right]_0^4$  **M1**  **A1**

   $\Rightarrow\ 4K - \dfrac{4}{3} = 1\ \Rightarrow\ K = \dfrac{1}{4}\left( 1 + \dfrac{4}{3} \right) = \dfrac{7}{12}.$  **A1**  **3 marks**

   (b) $\displaystyle\int_0^4 \left( \frac{7}{12}x - \frac{1}{16}x^3 \right) dx = \left[ \frac{7}{24}x^2 - \frac{1}{64}x^4 \right]_0^4$  **M1**  **A1**

   $\Rightarrow\ \left( \dfrac{7}{24} \times 16 - 4 \right) = \dfrac{14}{3} - 4 = \dfrac{2}{3}.$  **A1**

   $\Rightarrow$ Mean number of hours $= \dfrac{2}{3} \times 8 = 5\frac{1}{3}$  **B1**  **4 marks**

   (c) $P\,(>8\ \text{hours}) = \displaystyle\int_1^4 \left( \frac{7}{12} - \frac{x^2}{16} \right) dx = \left( \frac{7x}{12} - \frac{x^3}{48} \right)\Big]_1^4$  **M1**  **A1**

   $= \dfrac{28}{12} - \dfrac{4}{3} - \dfrac{7}{12} + \dfrac{1}{48} = \dfrac{21}{48} = \dfrac{7}{16}$  **A1**  **3 marks**

   (d) For f max. hours $= 4 \times 8 = 32 < 35.$  **B1**

   Also, radiation changes the form of the product.  **B1**  **2 marks**

   **TIP**

   Remember x is in units of 8 hours.

9. (a) $\lambda = 2.5$

   No faults $= e^{-2.5} = 0.0821.$  **M1**  **A1**  **2 marks**

   (b) 3 blankets. Average 2.5 faults $\Rightarrow\ \lambda = 7.5$  **M1**  **A1**

   Poisson $\Rightarrow\ e^{-7.5}\left( 1 + \dfrac{7.5}{1} + \dfrac{7.5^2}{1 \times 2} + \dfrac{7.5^3}{1 \times 2 \times 3} + \dfrac{7.5^4}{1 \times 2 \times 3 \times 4} + \cdots \right)$  **M1**  **A1**

   $P$ (No more than 4 faults)

   $= e^{-7.5}(1 + 7.5 + 28.125 + 70.3125 + 131.8936)$  **A2** (1,0)

   $\approx 0.1321 = 0.132.$  **6 marks**

   Normal distribution $(\lambda, \lambda)$

   $P\,(\leqslant 8.5)\quad P\left( Z < \dfrac{8.5 - 15}{\sqrt{15}} \right)$  **M1**  **A1**

   $\Rightarrow\ P < (-1.6783) = 1 - P(1.6783)$  **A1**

   $= 1 - 0.9533 = 0.0467$  **M1**

   $\approx 0.047.$  **A1**  **5 marks**

   **TIP**

   Remember a random variable $X \sim \text{Poi}(\lambda)$ can be approximated by $Y \sim N(\lambda, \lambda)$ for $\lambda > 10.$

**10.** (a)

| | | | | | | | | | | | | | | |
|---|---|---|---|---|---|---|---|---|---|---|---|---|---|---|
| 6 | 2 | 1 | 3 | 4 | 7 | 8 | 9 | | | | | | | 152 |
| 9 | 3 | 0 | 2 | 4 | 5 | 5 | 6 | 7 | 7 | 8 | | | | 314 |
| 13 | 4 | 1 | 2 | 3 | 3 | 4 | 4 | 5 | 5 | 5 | 6 | 7 | 8 | 8 | 581 |
| 7 | 5 | 1 | 2 | 4 | 4 | 6 | 7 | 8 | | | | | | 382 |
| 6 | 6 | 0 | 1 | 1 | 3 | 5 | 6 | | | | | | | 376 |
| 7 | 7 | 1 | 2 | 3 | 4 | 4 | 5 | 7 | | | | | | 516 |
| 3 | 8 | 0 | 2 | 4 | | | | | | | | | | 246 |
| $\overline{51}$ | | | | | | | | | | | | | | $\overline{2567}$    **B3** (2,1,0) |

$$\Rightarrow \text{Mean} = \frac{2567}{51} \approx 50.33 \quad \textbf{M1} \quad \textbf{A1}$$

$Q_1 = $ 13th Observation $= 37 \quad$ **M1**   **A1**

$Q_2 = $ 26th Observation $= 47$

$Q3 = $ 39th Observation $= 63 \quad$ **A1**    **8 marks**

(b)

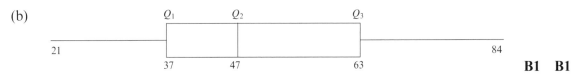

Slight positive skew.    **B1**    **3 marks**

(c)   Mode is 45.    $SIQR = \frac{1}{2}(63 - 37) = 13.$    **B1**   **M1**   **A1**     **3 marks**

> **TIP**
>
> Tabulate the marks in the stem and leaf diagram with inbuilt safety checks.

## Solutions to Paper 7 (Statistics)

**1.** (a)   Error is to reject the null hypothesis when it should have been accepted. Type I error.

                                                     **B1**     **1 mark**

(b)   Error is to accept the null hypothesis when it should have been rejected. Type II error.

                                                     **B1**     **1 mark**

(c)   To accept the null hypothesis when it should have been rejected. Type I error.

                                                     **B1**     **1 mark**

**2.** (a)   Mean weight $= \dfrac{7545}{150} = 50.3 \text{ kg}$    **M1**   **A1**

      Variance $\Rightarrow S^2 = \dfrac{381\,106 - 150 \times 50.3^2}{149} = 10.69$    **M1**   **A1**     **4 marks**

(b)   95% confidence interval for mean weight

      $\Rightarrow 50.3 \pm 1.96 \sqrt{\dfrac{10.69}{150}}$    **M1**   **A1**

      $\Rightarrow$ 49.78 to 50.82.    **A1**     **3 marks**

> **TIP**
>
> Remember the formulae for unbiased estimators of the mean and variance or know where to look them up in the formula booklet.

**3.** (a) Plot $y$ against $x$. **B2 B1 3 marks**

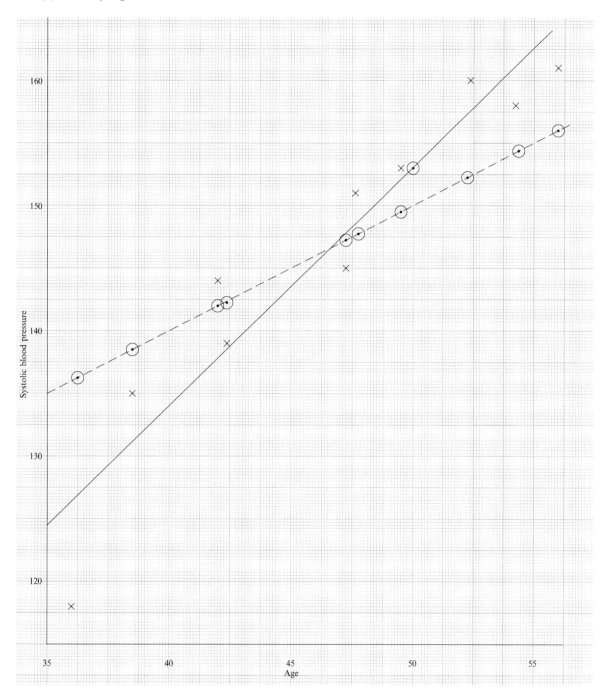

(b) Regression equation $y = mx + c$

$$m = \frac{n \sum xy - \sum x \cdot \sum y}{n \sum x^2 - (\sum x)^2} \quad \textbf{M1}$$

$$= \frac{689\,967 - 466.1 \times 1464}{221\,307.3 - 466.1^2} \approx 1.872. \quad \textbf{A1 A1}$$

$$c = \frac{\sum y}{n} - m \frac{\sum x}{n} = 146.4 - 1.872 \times 46.61 \quad \textbf{M1 A1}$$

$$\Rightarrow \quad c \approx 59.15$$

$$\Rightarrow \quad y = 1.872x + 59.15 \quad \textbf{A1} \qquad \textbf{6 marks}$$

(c)  The doctor's opinion is doubtful, as lines have quite different gradients (**B1**). However, beyond the age of around 47 these figures do possibly show increased stress causing increased blood pressure (**B1**).     **2 marks**

---

**TIP**

Do show all of your working to calculate the equation and do not just quote answers given by your calculator. An incorrect answer with no working does not get any marks.

---

**4.**  (a)  $\mu = np = \dfrac{100}{3}$     $\sigma^2 = npq = \dfrac{200}{9}$     **B1**  **B1**

$\Rightarrow\ Z = \dfrac{40 - \frac{1}{2} - 33.33}{\sqrt{\dfrac{200}{9}}} = 1.308$     **M1**  **A1**

$\Rightarrow\ P\,(\text{passing}) = 1 - 0.9046 = 0.0954$     **A1**     **5 marks**

(b)  $Z = \dfrac{39.5 - \dfrac{n}{3}}{\sqrt{\dfrac{2n}{9}}} = 1.645$     **A1**  **A1**  **B1**

$\Rightarrow\ 3\left(39.5 - \dfrac{n}{3}\right) = 1.645\sqrt{(2n)}.$

$118.5 - n = 1.645\sqrt{(2n)}.$

or    $(118.5 - n)^2 \equiv 5.412n$     **A1**

$\Rightarrow\ n^2 - (237 + 5.412)n + 14\,042.25 = 0$

$n = \frac{1}{2}[242.412 \pm \sqrt{(242.412^2 - 4 \times 14\,042.25)}]$     **M1**

$= 121.206 \pm 25.467 = 95.739\ (\text{or } 146.673)$     **A1**

$\Rightarrow$ Paper should contain a maximum of 95 questions.     **6 marks**

---

**TIP**

Remember $X \sim B(n, p)\ \Rightarrow\ Y \sim N(np, np(1 - p))$ and that as the normal distribution is a continuous distribution continuity corrections should be applied.

---

**5.**  (a)  Events occur at random in continuous time or space.     **B1**

Events occur singly and independently.     **B1**     **2 marks**

(b)  $\lambda = \dfrac{1}{104}(25 + 50 + 51 + 36 + 25) = 1.798 \approx 1.8$     **B1**  **1 mark**

(c)

| | | | Expected frequency | Observed | |
|---|---|---|---|---|---|
| 0 | $e^{-1.8}$ | $= 0.1653$ | 17.19 | 23 | |
| 1 | $1.8e^{-1.8}$ | $= 0.2975$ | 30.94 | 25 | **M1** |
| 2 | $\dfrac{1.8^2}{2!}e^{-1.8}$ | $= 0.2678$ | 27.85 | 25 | **A2** (1,0) |
| 3 | $\dfrac{1.8^3}{3!}e^{-1.8}$ | $= 0.1607$ | 16.71 | 17 | |

4   $\dfrac{1.8^4}{4!}e^{-1.8}$   $= 0.0723$ $\left.\right\}0.0983$   $7.52\left.\right\}10.22$   $9\left.\right\}14$

5   $\dfrac{1.8^5}{5!}e^{-1.8}$   $= 0.0260$   $2.70$   $5$   **M1**

$\dfrac{(O-E)^2}{e}$    1.9637, 1.1403, 0.2917, 0.0050, 1.3981

$\sum \dfrac{(O-E)^2}{E} = 4.7988$    **A1**

$H_0$ Breakdowns follow Poisson distribution with $\lambda = 1.8$.    **M1**

$H_1$ Breakdowns do not follow Poisson distribution with $\lambda = 1.8$.

Number of degrees of freedom $= 3$    **B1**

$\chi^2 = 7.81$    $4.7988 < 7.81$    **M1**

$\Rightarrow$ No evidence to reject $H_0$ at the 5% level

$\therefore$   Can be modelled by a Poisson distribution with $\lambda = 1.8$.    **A1**    **9 marks**

---

**TIP**

Make sure you know how to calculate (i) an estimate of the mean, (ii) the number of degrees of freedom and do state your null and alternative hypotheses. Do not forget to state your final conclusion.

---

6. (a)   Forming tree diagram    **M1   A1**

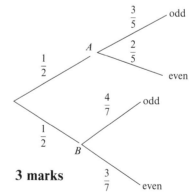

$P(\text{Even}) = \left(\dfrac{1}{2} \times \dfrac{2}{5} + \dfrac{1}{2} \times \dfrac{3}{7}\right)$    **M1   A1**

$= \dfrac{29}{70}$    **A1**    **5 marks**

(b)   $P(\text{Box } A) = \dfrac{\dfrac{1}{2} \times \dfrac{3}{5}}{\left(\dfrac{1}{2} \times \dfrac{3}{5} + \dfrac{1}{2} \times \dfrac{4}{7}\right)} = \dfrac{21}{41}$    **M1   A1   A1**    **3 marks**

(c)   $P(E + O \text{ Box } A) = 2\left[\left(\dfrac{1}{2} \times \dfrac{2}{5}\right) \times \left(\dfrac{1}{2} \times \dfrac{3}{4}\right)\right]$   or   $2\left[\left(\dfrac{1}{2} \times \dfrac{3}{5}\right) \times \left(\dfrac{1}{2} \times \dfrac{2}{4}\right)\right]$    **M1   A1**

$= \dfrac{3}{20}$

$P(E + O \text{ Box } B) = 2\left[\left(\dfrac{1}{2} \times \dfrac{3}{7}\right) \times \left(\dfrac{1}{2} \times \dfrac{4}{6}\right)\right] = \dfrac{1}{7}$

$$P\begin{pmatrix} E \text{ Box } B + O \text{ Box } A \\ \text{or} \\ O \text{ Box } A + E \text{ Box } B \end{pmatrix} = 2\left[\left(\frac{1}{2} \times \frac{3}{7}\right) \times \left(\frac{1}{2} \times \frac{3}{5}\right)\right] = \frac{9}{70} \quad \textbf{A2} \ (1,0)$$

$$P\begin{pmatrix} O \text{ Box } B + E \text{ Box } A \\ \text{or} \\ E \text{ Box } A + O \text{ Box } B \end{pmatrix} = 2\left[\left(\frac{1}{2} \times \frac{4}{7}\right) \times \left(\frac{1}{2} \times \frac{2}{5}\right)\right] = \frac{4}{35}$$

$$P(\text{One odd, one even}) = \frac{3}{20} + \frac{1}{7} + \frac{9}{70} + \frac{4}{35} = \frac{75}{140} = \frac{15}{28} \quad \textbf{A1} \qquad \textbf{5 marks}$$

**TIP**

Show clearly the probabilities on the tree diagram.

7.  (a)  $\hat{p} = \dfrac{60}{90} = \dfrac{2}{3}$ **B1**

$$\Rightarrow \frac{2}{3} - 1.96\sqrt{\frac{\frac{2}{3}\left(1 - \frac{2}{3}\right)}{90}} < p < \frac{2}{3} + 1.96\sqrt{\frac{\frac{2}{3}\left(1 - \frac{2}{3}\right)}{90}} \quad \textbf{M1}$$

$$\Rightarrow \quad 0.5693 < p < 0.7641 \quad \textbf{A1} \quad \textbf{A1}$$

Is approximate since we have used $\hat{p} = \dfrac{2}{3}$. **B1** **5 marks**

(b)  For large $n_1$, $n_2$.    $N\left(p_1 - p_2, \dfrac{p_1q_1}{90} + \dfrac{p_2q_2}{80}\right)$ **B1** **B1**

$H_0$: $p_1 - p_2 = 0$    $H_1$: $p_1 - p_2 \neq 0$ **M1**

$$Z = \frac{\dfrac{2}{3} - \dfrac{5}{8}}{\sqrt{\dfrac{\frac{2}{3} \times \frac{1}{3}}{90} + \dfrac{\frac{5}{8} \times \frac{3}{8}}{80}}} = \frac{\dfrac{1}{24}}{\sqrt{\dfrac{2}{810} + \dfrac{15}{5120}}} \approx 0.567 \quad \textbf{M1} \quad \textbf{A1} \quad \textbf{A1}$$

Critical region $z \leqslant -1.645$ or $\geqslant 1.645$ **B1**

$\therefore$ Cannot reject $H_0 \Rightarrow$ No evidence of a difference between the effectiveness of the two drugs. **A1** **8 marks**

**TIP**

For large $n_1$, $n_2$    $N\left(p_1 - p_2, \dfrac{p_1q_1}{n_1} + \dfrac{p_2q_2}{n_2}\right)$.

8.  (a)  None in favour $= \left(\dfrac{3}{4}\right)^6$    One in favour $= 6\left(\dfrac{3}{4}\right)^5\left(\dfrac{1}{4}\right)$ **B1** **B1**

Probability at least 2 in favour $= 1 - (0.178 + 0.356)$ **M1**

$$= 0.466 \quad \textbf{A1} \qquad \textbf{4 marks}$$

(b)  $N\left(250 \times \dfrac{1}{4}, 250 \times \dfrac{1}{4} \times \dfrac{3}{4}\right) = N(62.5, 46.875)$ **B1** **B1**

$$\Phi \Rightarrow \frac{44.5 - 62.5}{\sqrt{46.875}} = \Phi(-2.629) \quad \textbf{M1} \quad \textbf{A1}$$

$$\Phi \Rightarrow \frac{70.5 - 62.5}{\sqrt{46.875}} = \Phi(1.168) \quad \textbf{A1}$$

$$\Rightarrow -\Phi(-2.629) + \Phi(1.168) = 0.8786 - (1 - 0.9957) \quad \textbf{M1}$$

$$= 0.8786 - 0.0043 = 0.8743. \quad \textbf{A1} \qquad \textbf{7 marks}$$

(c) $\dfrac{\dfrac{45}{200} - 0.25}{\sqrt{\dfrac{0.25 \times 0.75}{200}}} \approx -0.8165$  **M1**

$H_0$: $p = 0.25$,  $H_1$: $p < 0.25$  **M1**

$\Phi(-0.8165) = 1 - 0.7930 = 0.207 > 0.05$  **A1**

$\therefore$ Cannot reject $H_0$ and Editor is correct in claiming 25% support for the new format.

**A1    4 marks**

> **TIP**
>
> Remember $Y \sim N(np, np(1-p))$ and that continuity corrections are required.

**9.**

|         | Recover | Not recover |     |
|---------|---------|-------------|-----|
| A Serum | 65      | 15          | 80  |
| B Serum | 80      | 40          | 120 |
|         | 145     | 55          | 200 |

**B2** $(1, 0)$

|   | Recover | Not recover |     |
|---|---------|-------------|-----|
| A | $\dfrac{80 \times 145}{200} = 58$ | 22 | 80 |
| B | 87 | 33 | 120 |
|   | 145 | 55 | 200 |

**M1  A1  A1**

**A1  A1**

| Observed | Estimate | $O - E - \frac{1}{2}$ | $(\lvert O - E \rvert - \frac{1}{2})^2$ |
|----------|----------|------------------------|------------------------------------------|
| 65 | 58 | $6\frac{1}{2}$ | 0.7284 |
| 80 | 87 | $6\frac{1}{2}$ | 0.4856 |
| 15 | 22 | $6\frac{1}{2}$ | 1.9205 |
| 40 | 33 | $6\frac{1}{2}$ | 1.2803 |
|    |    |                | 4.4148 |

**M1**

**A1**

**A1**

$H_0$: Treatment has no effect.  **B1**

$H_1$: Treatment is effective.  **B1**

Degree of freedom $\nu = 1$.

$4.4148 > 3.841$:  Reject $H_0$ at 5% level $\Rightarrow$ Effective  **M1  A1**

$< 5.024$:  Accept $H_0$ at 2.5% level $\Rightarrow$ Not effective.  **A1    15 marks**

> **TIP**
>
> Set out your working clearly in tabular form and show how you have arrived at your figures.

## Solutions to Paper 8 (Statistics)

**1.** (a) $K + 8K + 27K + 64K = 1 \Rightarrow K = \dfrac{1}{100}$  **B1    1 mark**

(b) $E(X) = (1 + 16 + 81 + 256)K \Rightarrow E(X) = \dfrac{354}{100} = 3.54$  **M1  A1**

$$\text{Var}(X) = (1 + 32 + 243 + 1024)K - 3.54^2 = 0.4684 \approx 0.47 \quad \textbf{M1} \quad \textbf{A1} \qquad \textbf{4 marks}$$

(c) $E(4X - 5) = 4E(X) - 5 = 4 \times 3.54 - 5 = 9.16$ **M1** **A1**

$\text{Var}(4X - 5) = 16\,\text{Var}(X) = 16 \times 0.4684 \approx 7.49$ **B1** **3 marks**

---

**TIP**

Remember $\sum P(X) = 1$, $E(aX + b) = aE(X) + b$, $\text{Var}(aX + b) = a^2 V(X)$.

---

2. (a) $4 \times (0.25)^3(0.75) = 0.046875 \approx 0.0469$ **M1** **A1** **2 marks**

(b) $0.984$ **B1** **1 mark**

(c) $0.15 \times 0.25 + 0.85 \times 0.05 = 0.08$ **M1** **A1** **A1** **3 marks**

(d) $P(\text{Ann}|\text{Error}) = \dfrac{0.15 \times 0.25}{0.08} = 0.46875$ **A1**

$P(\text{Jean}|\text{Error}) = \dfrac{0.85 \times 0.05}{0.08} = 0.53125$ **M1** **A1**

$P(\text{Ann}|\text{Error}) \bigcap P(\text{Jean}|\text{Error}) = 2 \times 0.46875 \times 0.53125$

$\approx 0.498 \approx 0.50$ **A1** **4 marks**

---

**TIP**

Make sure you understand conditional probability

$P(A|B) = \dfrac{P(A \bigcap B)}{P(B)}$.

---

3. (a) $\sum X = 4 \qquad \sum Y = 6.27$ **B1** **B1**

$$r = \frac{\sum XY - \frac{1}{6}\sum X \cdot \sum Y}{\left[\left(\sum X^2 - \frac{(\sum X)^2}{6}\right)\left(\sum Y^2 - \frac{(\sum Y)^2}{6}\right)\right]^{\frac{1}{2}}} \quad \textbf{M1}$$

$$= \frac{4.4029 - 4.19045}{\left[\left(2.9144 - \frac{4^2}{6}\right)\left(6.7871 - \frac{6.27^2}{6}\right)\right]^{\frac{1}{2}}} \quad \textbf{A1}$$

$\approx 0.924$ **A1** **5 marks**

(b)

| Ranks | 1 | 2 | 3 | 4 | 5 | 6 | |
|-------|---|---|---|---|---|---|---|
| X | 2 | 5 | 4 | 6 | 3 | 1 | **M1** |
| Y | 3 | 6 | 4 | 5 | 2 | 1 | |
| $d^2$ | 1 | 1 | 0 | 1 | 1 | 0 | **A1** |

$\Rightarrow r_s = 1 - \dfrac{6\sum d^2}{n(n^2 - 1)} = 1 - \dfrac{6 \times 4}{6 \times 35} = 0.8857$ **M1** **A1**

$\Rightarrow r_s \approx 0.886$ **A1** **5 marks**

---

**TIP**

Remember your formulae for the product moment correlation coefficient and the Spearman Rank correlation coefficient.

**4.** (a)  Standard Error of mean $= \dfrac{\sigma}{\sqrt{n}} = \dfrac{0.1}{\sqrt{100}} = 0.01$  **M1  A1**

$z = \dfrac{|1.5421| - 1.5}{0.01} = 2.4$  **M1  A1**

$H_0$: $\mu = 1.5$  $H_1$: $\mu \neq 1.5$  Two-tailed  **M1  A1**

Critical Value at 1% level $= 2.576$  **B1**

$2.4 < 2.576 \Rightarrow$ cannot reject $H_0$  **A1**

$\Rightarrow$ Accept $H_0$ and conclude overall mean weight is 1.5 kg.  **8 marks**

(b)  $H_0$: $\mu = 1.5$  $H_1$: $\mu < 1.5$  One-tailed.  **M1**

Only significant if $z < -2.323$  $\therefore$  Accept $H_0$

$\Rightarrow$ No evidence that $\mu < 1.5$ kg.  **A1**  **2 marks**

---

**TIP**

Remember $SE_x = \dfrac{\sigma}{\sqrt{n}}$. State your hypotheses and conclusions.

---

**5.** (a)  $t = 15$  $\mu = \dfrac{15}{125} = 0.12$.  **B1**

$P(>2) = 1 - [P(0) + P(1) + P(2)] = 1 - e^{-0.12}(1 + 0.12 + \frac{1}{2}(0.12)^2)$  **M1  A1**

$= 1 - 0.999737 \approx 0.000263$  **A1**  **4 marks**

(b)  $e^{-0.008t} = 0.95 \Rightarrow -0.008t = \ln(0.95)$  **M1  A1**

$= t = \dfrac{1}{0.008}\left(\ln \dfrac{1}{0.95}\right) \approx 6.41 = 6$ mins.  **A1**  **3 marks**

(c)  $t = 12\frac{1}{2}$ hrs $\Rightarrow \mu = \dfrac{12.5 \times 60}{125} = 6$.  **B1**

$H_0$: $\mu = 6$  $H_1$: $\mu < 6$  **M1**

$P(\geqslant 9) = 1 - P(\leqslant 8) = 1 - 0.847 = 0.153 > 0.05$  **A1**

$\Rightarrow$ Cannot reject $H_0 \Rightarrow$ Conclude there is no evidence to suggest the mean has changed.  **A1**  **4 marks**

---

**TIP**

$P(n > 2) = 1 - [P(n = 0) + P(n = 1) + P(n = 2)]$

Remember that cumulative Poisson Probability tables are usually for $P(X \leqslant Y)$ and not $P(X < Y)$.

---

**6.** (a)  $P_1 = \dfrac{198}{900} = 0.22$  $P_2 = \dfrac{150}{600} = 0.25$  **B1**

$H_0$: $\mu_2 = \mu_1$  $H_1$: $\mu_2 > \mu_1$  One-tailed  **M1**  **2 marks**

(b)  Pooled $P = \dfrac{198 + 150}{900 + 600} = \dfrac{348}{1500} = 0.232$  **M1  A1**

$\Rightarrow q = 1 - P = 1 - 0.232 = 0.768$  **A1**

$\sqrt{\left[\dfrac{0.232 \times 0.768}{900} + \dfrac{0.232 \times 0.768}{600}\right]} = 0.02225$  **M1  A1**

$z = \dfrac{0.22 - 0.25}{0.02225} = 1.348$  **M1  A1**

Critical value at 5% level $= 1.64 > 1.348$    **M1**

$\Rightarrow$ Insufficient evidence to reject $H_0$.    **M1**

Conclude that number of people knowing of 'Improved Brand X' is the same.

**9 marks**

7.

|  | For the motion | Against the motion | Undecided |  |
|---|---|---|---|---|
| **Girls** | 98  (85.64) | 42  (51.49) | 15  (17.86) | 155 |
| **Boys** | 65  (77.36) | 56  (46.51) | 19  (16.14) | 140 |
|  | 163 | 98 | 34 | 295 |

**M1**

**A4** (3,2,1,0)

| Observed | Estimated | $\dfrac{(O - E)^2}{E}$ |
|---|---|---|
| 98 | 85.64 | 1.78 |
| 42 | 51.49 | 1.75 |
| 15 | 17.86 | 0.46 |
| 65 | 77.36 | 1.97 |
| 56 | 46.51 | 1.94 |
| 19 | 16.14 | 0.51 |
|  |  | 8.41 |

**M1**    **A3** $(2, 1, 0)$

$H_0$: No difference of opinion.

$H_1$: Difference of opinion.    **M1**

The degrees of freedom $= 2 \times 1 = 2$.    **B1**

Significant level at 5% $= 5.991 < 8.41$    **M1**

$\Rightarrow$ Reject $H_0$ and accept $H_1$ i.e. there is a difference of opinion between boys and girls as far as the proposal is concerned.    **A1**    **13 marks**

**TIP**

To maximise your marks make sure you show all of your working so that the examiner knows exactly what method you are using.

8.

| Mid-points | 152.5 | 157.5 | 162.5 | 167.5 | 172.5 | 177.5 | 182.5 | 187.5 | 192.5 | 197.5 |
|---|---|---|---|---|---|---|---|---|---|---|
| Frequency | 2 | 5 | 4 | 9 | 20 | 12 | 9 | 7 | 3 | 1 |

**M1**

(a)    $\Rightarrow$ Mean height $= \dfrac{12\,560}{72} = 174.4$ cm.    **A1**    **2 marks**

(b)    $\sum f(x - \bar{x})^2 \Rightarrow$ Variance $\dfrac{6877.92}{72} \approx 95.5$    **M1**

Standard deviation $\sqrt{95.5} \approx 9.77$.    **A1**    **2 marks**

(c)  Upper class boundaries  155  160  165  170  175  180  185  190  195  200

Cumulative totals      2    7    11   20   40   52   61   68   71   72

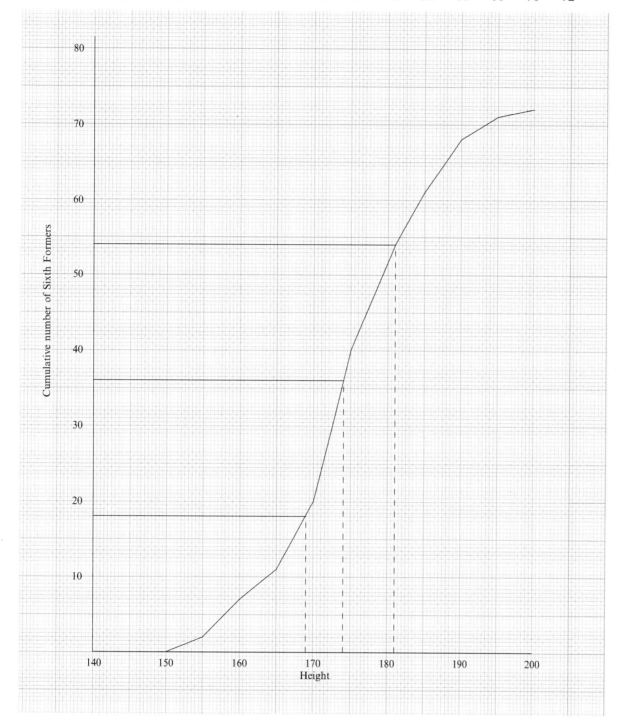

**M1  A1    2 marks**

(d)  Median mark 174.0    **B1**

$Q_1 = 169.0$, $Q_3 = 181.0$    **B1**

$Q_3 - Q_2 = 7.0$, $Q_2 - Q_1 = 5.0$    **B1**

$\Rightarrow \; Q_2 - Q_1 < Q_3 - Q_2 \; \Rightarrow$ Positive skew.    **B1**    **4 marks**

(e)  All Sixth Formers $\hat{\mu} = 174.4$,    $\hat{\sigma}^2 = \dfrac{6877.92}{71} = 96.87$    **B1  M1  A1    3 marks**

**TIP**

Do not forget to plot the cumulative frequencies on the graph at the upper class limits of the class to which they refer.

**9.** (a) $\dfrac{1}{18} a \cdot 3^2 - \dfrac{1}{27} \cdot 3^3 = 1 \Rightarrow a = 4.$     **M1   A1       2 marks**

(b) $\dfrac{dF}{dx} = \dfrac{1}{18} \cdot 4 \cdot 2x - \dfrac{1}{27} \cdot 3x^2 \Rightarrow$ f$(x) = 0, \qquad x < 0$     **M1   A1**

$$= \dfrac{4}{9} \cdot x - \dfrac{1}{9} \cdot x^2, \qquad 0 \leqslant x \leqslant 3 \qquad \textbf{A1}$$

$$= 0, \qquad x > 3. \qquad \textbf{3 marks}$$

(c) $\dfrac{df}{dx} = \dfrac{4}{9} - \dfrac{2}{9} \cdot x = 0 \qquad x = 2 \Rightarrow$ Modal value $x = 2.$     **B1     1 mark**

(d) Median $m$ is given by $\dfrac{2}{9} m^2 - \dfrac{1}{27} m^3 = \dfrac{1}{2} \Rightarrow 2m^3 - 12m^2 + 27 = 0$     **M1   A1**

f$(1.8) = -0.216,$ f$(1.79) = +0.0214 \Rightarrow$ changes sign

$\Rightarrow$ median between 1.79 and 1.80     **A1     3 marks**

(e) $E(X) = \displaystyle\int_0^3 x \left( \dfrac{4x}{9} - \dfrac{1}{9} x^2 \right) dx = \left[ \dfrac{4}{27} x^3 - \dfrac{1}{36} x^4 \right]_0^3 = \dfrac{7}{4}.$     **M1   A1**

$E(X^2) = \displaystyle\int_0^3 x^2 \left( \dfrac{4x}{9} - \dfrac{1}{9} x^2 \right) dx = \left[ \dfrac{4}{9} \cdot \dfrac{x^4}{4} - \dfrac{x^5}{45} \right]_0^3 = 3\dfrac{3}{5}$     **M1   A1**

$\therefore \quad \text{Var}(X) = 3\dfrac{3}{5} - \left( \dfrac{7}{4} \right)^2 = 3\dfrac{3}{5} - 3\dfrac{1}{16} = \dfrac{43}{80}.$     **A1     5 marks**

**TIP**

Do not mix up the cumulative distribution function $F(x)$ with the probability density function f$(x)$. Remember

$$\dfrac{dF(x)}{dx} = f(x).$$